Special Praise for *Lo...*

"In the daunting face of a rising epidemic of depression, addiction, and suicide, Dr Hill's personal story emerges as a touchstone of essential wisdom in how to address such hardships, energized by compassionate healing. This book is a wakeup call, not only for the medical profession, but for our culture at large. Such profound healing indeed offers great hope, and is best achieved through the sage and honest application of empathy and compassion based on our shared nature and purpose."

—Eben Alexander, MD
Neurosurgeon and bestselling author of *Living in a Mindful Universe* and *Proof of Heaven*

"Dr. Adam Hill tells a powerfully compelling narrative of a riveting journey, uniquely his and yet with universal insights shared by all healers who have suffered—and isn't that all of us? The reader is given a window into the inner world of vulnerability, self-doubt, and struggle, juxtaposed with the external facade of toughness that can erode our greatest tools—empathy for others and compassion for our own imperfections. Exposing the stigmatizing and illogical aspects of the culture of medicine when it comes to caring for our own, this book has the power to transform an already shifting culture and should be required reading for all professionals in the medical field."

—Christine Moutier, MD
Chief Medical Officer, American Foundation for Suicide Prevention

"I did not need to read this book to be able to describe the incredible integrity and merits of Dr. Adam Hill. I've had the honor of working with him on some very difficult cases over the years. Reading the book, however, gives one the insight necessary to gain an understanding of the suffering Adam endured in a way that, hopefully, will help others in the same boat. In reading his words, he is both the fragile man in the book and the amazing man that he has become in recovery. His transparency and integrity will undoubtedly help reduce fear associated with being honest. His commitment to reduce stigma and embrace being a flawed human being as we all are is an example for us all. Thank you, Adam, for the courage and the reminder!"

—**Jim Ryser, MA, LMHC, LCAC, TTS**
Chronic Pain and Addiction Specialist
Former Arista Records solo artist and guitarist for John Mellencamp

"Although about addiction and depression, this is a hope-filled book that speaks directly to those overworked, over-committed, and 'burned out.' Dr. Hill is the prototypical 'wounded healer' whose life story exemplifies that in helping others reciprocal healing occurs. For those feeling helpless and hopeless, this book can be life-saving."

—**Joseph Maroon, MD**
Professor of Neurosurgery and Heindl Scholar in Neuroscience
University of Pittsburgh Medical Center
Author of *Square One: The Secret to a Balanced Life*

"There's no healing without connection, no matter how much we want it to be otherwise. This is the very honest, unadorned story of a young man who wants to be a doctor without quite knowing why and who cracks up on the rocks of self-will, depression, and addiction. He very nearly drowns, but happily for him, for his patients, and the rest of us, he does not. He survives and learns how to use his suffering for his own and the greater good, and for more connection, less isolation, and more healing. Thank you, Adam."

—**Mark Vonnegut, MD**

"Adam Hill has given us an extraordinary gift. Yes, Dr. Hill is a natural storyteller and the writing is beautiful. Yes, the observations he makes about the isolation of physicians struggling in a system that despises weakness are astonishing and desperately needed. And yes, his suggestions for transforming the culture of medicine, which has grown so ill, are among the wisest and most insightful words on the topic I have read in a decade. These are all gifts, and we should be deeply grateful to him. But the truly extraordinary gift he has given us is the gift of his own honesty and vulnerability. He has offered a hope that heals to those of us who have struggled with depression, addiction, anxiety, or the lonely fear that so many of us experience in the journey called 'becoming a doctor.' By opening himself to us, he has shown us a way out of the woods. I wish every medical student, resident, and attending physician in the country had a copy of this extraordinary book."

—Raymond Barfield, MD, PhD
Professor of Pediatrics and Christian Philosophy, Duke University

"*Long Walk Out of the Woods* is a memoir of addiction and redemption told with self-awareness, humility, and candor. Dr. Hill exposes the professional obstacles that doctors experience when they seek help for depression and substance use."

—Dr. Judy Melinek
Coauthor of *Working Stiff: Two Years, 262 Bodies,*
and the Making of a Medical Examiner

"Stigma is a formidable barrier to mental healthcare. Consequently, despite the availability of effective treatment, many people with mental health difficulties, especially physicians, continue to suffer in silence. Dr. Adam Hill's candid and courageous account of his lived experience as a doctor who recovered from a mental health condition is a watershed moment in medicine and will undoubtedly help to combat stigma and discrimination and break down the barriers to mental healthcare for those who urgently need it. *Long Walk Out of the Woods* traces Dr. Hill's inspirational recovery journey. His moving story will make you cry tears of joy and sorrow and will provide you with a precious insight into the heart and mind of an extraordinary man."

—Ahmed Hankir, MD
Royal College of Psychiatrists award-winning
doctor and author of *The Wounded Healer*

Long Walk
Out *of the* Woods

Long Walk
Out *of the* Woods

A PHYSICIAN'S STORY OF ADDICTION, DEPRESSION, HOPE, AND RECOVERY

ADAM B. HILL

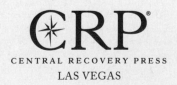

CENTRAL RECOVERY PRESS
LAS VEGAS

Central Recovery Press (CRP) is committed to publishing exceptional materials addressing addiction treatment, recovery, and behavioral healthcare topics.

For more information, visit www.centralrecoverypress.com.

Publisher: Central Recovery Press
            3321 N. Buffalo Drive
            Las Vegas, NV 89129

24 23 22 21 20 19   1 2 3 4 5

Library of Congress Cataloging-in-Publication Data

Names: Hill, Adam B., author.
Title: Long walk out of the woods : a physician's story of addiction,
    depression, hope, and recovery / Adam B. Hill.
Description: Las Vegas : Central Recovery Press, 2019.
Identifiers: LCCN 2019026053 (print) | LCCN 2019026054 (ebook) | ISBN
    9781949481228 (trade paperback) | ISBN 9781949481235 (ebook)
Subjects: LCSH: Hill, Adam B.--Mental health. | Physicians--United
    States--Biography. | Recovering alcoholics--United States--Biography. |
    Physicians--Mental health. | Burn out (Psychology)
Classification: LCC RC451.4.P5 H55 2019 (print) | LCC RC451.4.P5 (ebook)
    | DDC 610.92 [B]--dc23
LC record available at https://lccn.loc.gov/2019026053
LC ebook record available at https://lccn.loc.gov/2019026054

Photo of Adam B. Hill used with permission of Indiana University School of Medicine.

Every attempt has been made to contact copyright holders. If copyright holders have not been properly acknowledged, please contact us. Central Recovery Press will be happy to rectify the omission in future printings of this book.

Publisher's Note: This book contains general information about addiction, recovery, and related matters. The information is not medical advice. This book is not an alternative to medical advice from your doctor or other professional healthcare provider.

Our books represent the experiences and opinions of their authors only. Every effort has been made to ensure that events, institutions, and statistics presented in our books as facts are accurate and up-to-date. To protect their privacy, the names of some of the people, places, and institutions in this book may have been changed.

Cover and interior design and layout by Deb Tremper, Six Penny Graphics

To all of those people still suffering in silence,

and to those who helped me find my own voice.

Table of Contents

Preface

My name is Adam. I'm a human being, husband, father, physician, recovering alcoholic, and mental health patient. After struggling with depression for years, I drank away the mounting problems in my life, one night and one bottle at a time. Debilitating consumption became commonplace as I spiraled deeper into the recesses of active addiction. And in those depths, I searched for any possible way for the ongoing pain to end.

In the midst of these struggles, working in modern medicine fractured my identity, stole my authenticity, and left me a shell of the person I wanted to be. I had dedicated my life to medicine, but when my own life hung in the balance, medicine turned a blind eye to my suffering.

I risk everything in telling this story—my career, livelihood, and reputation—but I feel there is no other way forward. It's time for my voice to be heard. In this book, I chronicle addiction, depression, and suicidal plans in the same context, because they all overlapped in my life. However, I don't wish to suggest a direct causal relationship between addiction, mental health conditions, and suicide. Each issue is complex, unique, and often difficult to fully understand. Untreated mental health conditions do contribute to increased risks of suicide. Substance use is a common means of self-medication for mental health conditions, and for some individuals substance use evolves into active addiction. But suicide is a more complex cultural phenomenon than can be explained by simple associations with mental health and/or substance use.

I write this book in the face of a national epidemic of suicide, and amidst a widespread neglect of mental health conditions for people working in medicine. The overall suicide rate in the United States has increased 25 percent over the past twenty years.[1] In diverse groups such as millennials, veterans, farmers, teenagers, and the elderly, suicide rates continue to surge. The average number of teenage males dying by suicide increased 30 percent between 2007–2015. During the same time period, suicide rates among female teens nearly doubled, reaching a forty-year high.[2] Veterans, a group comprising 8.5 percent of the US population, account for a staggering 18 percent of adult suicides.[3] Yet the highest suicide rates don't exist within the military community, as people sometimes assume. The highest suicide rate within any profession exists in the medical field.

Every year in this country, approximately 400 physicians take their own lives, a rate two times higher than the national average.[4] That means entire classes worth of medical school students vanish due to suicide in what has become a hidden mental health crisis. Broken systems, neglect, fear, and judgment are partially to blame. Current studies report that more than 50 percent of medical professionals show signs of distress, with rising levels of compassion fatigue, apathy, and untreated mental health conditions.[5,6] Yet the medical community's system and culture encourage secrecy when seeking mental health treatment. The ostracization of professionals living with these conditions reflects a culture that still stigmatizes the estimated 20 percent of Americans who live with mental health conditions. The truth is, a striking majority of medical professionals don't seek help because of the fearful culture we created ourselves. In perpetuating this problem, we set a tragic and horrifying example for the people under our care.

While traveling the country in preparation for this book, I found that in some circles, public perceptions of mental health conditions are still limited to straitjackets, lobotomies, padded rooms, and tinfoil hats. The "mental illness" portrayed on the big screen often involves locked institutions, crazed gunmen, psychopaths, or mass murderers. I fear we continue to equate mental health conditions with incompetence or irrational and illogical thoughts that lead to deviant behaviors, which promotes fear-based reactions when someone shares that a medical professional is afflicted by a mental condition. Such knee-jerk reactions proclaim individuals to be unfit, unreliable, and ill equipped to hold such a skill-oriented and knowledge-based position.

In 2017, the United States National Institute of Mental Health revealed that 19 percent of adults over eighteen years of age had been diagnosed with a mental health condition.[7] The World Health Organization estimates that 450 million people are affected by mental health conditions globally, making these ailments the leading cause of illness in the world.[8] And worldwide, evidence continues to show that worsening mental health is an occupational work hazard in the medical field.

I know firsthand how much one's mental health can deteriorate during medical training. Studies have shown that 27 percent of medical students are depressed, a rate three times higher than an aged-matched cohort of their peers.[9] The numbers don't get any better after graduation either, as depression rates among medical residents are an estimated 29 percent.[10] In medical schools in the United Kingdom, a multi-school study found 52 percent of medical students reported substantial levels of anxiety.[11] While another study found the proportion of medical interns meeting criteria for depression increased from a baseline of 3.9 percent prior to medical training to a staggering 25.7 percent during medical internship.[12] In the group of individuals reporting their mental health conditions, more than 80 percent did not feel adequately supported in their disclosure.[13] The substance use rates for veterinarians, dentists, nurses, and physicians hover around the national average of 10 to 12 percent, but some researchers believe those numbers are underreported and may in fact be as high as

15 to 20 percent.[14-15, 25-26] And, as with myself, over 10 million people in the United States have coexisting mental health and addiction stories.[16]

These numbers are often used to scare people into default assumptions about the quality of medical care delivered by professionals with mental health conditions. We are conditioned to think stereotypically about mental health, but medical professionals are human beings too, and these conditions are treatable. In addiction treatment for professionals, some programs report up to 90 percent five-year sobriety rates, a number astoundingly higher than national treatment averages.[17-20] With medication, counseling, and/or tailored treatment plans, the vast majority of individuals with mental health and/or addiction conditions remain incredibly reliable and productive in their work. Despite common misperceptions, physicians with a mental health and/or addiction condition, while in a professional treatment program, are actually 20 percent *less* likely to have a malpractice lawsuit filed against them than their peers.[21] Most of the time no one would even know they have a history of any mental health condition. In fact, some of your favorite doctors, nurses, and therapists likely have a mental health past, and it should not be an indictment of them. These individuals often provide more compassionate care because they understand what it feels like to be sick. This is not a flaw; it's actually a gift.

The presence of these conditions alone should not scare anyone, but the increasing incidence of mental health conditions, the rising rates of suicide, and the infrequency with which medical professionals seek treatment should alarm us all. In one study, Dr. Katherine Gold found that 50 percent of physicians reported signs or symptoms of a mental health condition but did not seek treatment for it.[6] Another study showed medical school students are less likely to seek treatment than the general population despite having better access to care.[22] In both studies, stigma and a fear of potential repercussions for their careers were identified as the biggest barriers to seeking treatment. This fear of repercussions is not unwarranted, as a significant number of state medical licensing boards, hospitals, and insurance malpractice carriers require medical professionals to disclose their mental health treatment histories when applying for jobs. Downstream, because this fear-based work culture dissuades individuals from seeking appropriate mental health care, people work sicker, while being subjected to increased workplace demands in the rapidly shifting bureaucratic business of modern medicine, with less professional autonomy and more feelings of helplessness. In the end, the cumulative effects all contribute to a suicide rate that has reached epidemic levels.

I acknowledge that there is a shortage of mental health resources in this country. A conservative estimate shows 44 percent of individuals living with mental health conditions do not or cannot receive adequate, timely, and/or affordable services. In countries with less developed resources, that number may be as high as 90 percent.[23] The fact is, the United States' healthcare system is ineffective, inaccessible, and unaffordable for a significant portion of the population, which leads to enormous amounts of harm. Year after year, nearly 65 percent of US bankruptcy claims are secondary to medical debt.[24] Despite efforts to improve access to healthcare through the Affordable Care Act and Mental Health Parity Act, a significant amount of people with medical insurance remain poorly covered when it comes to mental health services. I know that implicit biases and explicit treatment barriers based on gender, race, sexual orientation, ethnicity, and religion often stand in the way of adequate treatment. I've also seen disparities, injustices, and indignities in the legal system that criminalize both mental health and addiction. I don't pretend to know what it's like to live with different medical conditions, under different circumstances, in a different skin, or with obstacles that are different than my own. As a white, upper-middle-class American with an in-demand career, I've been afforded opportunities and access to resources unavailable to a majority of people. I think it best to acknowledge that up front. But I do come from humble beginnings, and I learned at an early age that every individual's story matters, so I work diligently in medicine to bring about change and expand opportunities for all people to get the help they deserve. I can't imagine what another person's life is like, but I continue to listen and to learn from other people's perspectives.

In writing this book, I wish to be part of a larger solution that will help improve access, treatment options, and resources for all people affected by mental health conditions, not just individuals working in medicine, because real human beings exist within all these statistical percentiles. Every day, people die because we accept or are complicit in a system that allows individuals with mental health conditions to be subjected to punishment, stigma, blame, and retribution for seeking help for treatable problems. The statistics I've shared are about as academic as this book gets. It's not my intent to present a scholarly examination of this ongoing epidemic, filled with articles, charts, and graphs. Several colleagues have dedicated their careers to dissecting these issues scientifically, and their work is invaluable. Mine is but a reflection on my personal experience living with mental health conditions while working in modern medicine.

I hope to provide insight into what it feels like to live with these conditions in personal and professional worlds that attach shame to their very existence. I write from a standpoint of vulnerable truth, hoping to shed light on an evolving epidemic both in healthcare and in our culture at large. Intimate details from the formative years of my early childhood to an emerging medical career that was plagued by addiction and depression will be shared. And I'll go not only into the depths of my disease, but also share lessons learned in my years of recovery. Some of the stories are emotional, tragic, and unsettling, but I believe they're all worth telling. To offer additional perspectives, I'll also share stories from other individuals with mental health conditions, and those of patients under my care. To respect their privacy and in compliance with medical regulations, names, diagnoses, parts of the stories, and other identifying information have been changed, with the exception of a few people who wished for their unedited story to be told.

I share these stories as a survivor, and because something must be done to confront this deadly culture. I hope this book serves as a testimony to the power of authentically sharing our own stories, because ultimately I want other people to know they're not alone. No one should have to walk fearfully on the lonely road toward seeking assistance for these treatable conditions. I write to encourage lifting the mental health shroud to reveal positive role models, an effort to lead us all out of the darkness and into the light.

No one is on this journey alone—I promise you.

I know what it feels like to be isolated in these conditions. I know what it feels like to accept your own death as the only means of escape. And I've lost six beloved colleagues to suicide since I started my career in medicine, some of whom, like myself, struggled with depression and addiction, while others battled obsessive-compulsive disorder (OCD), post-traumatic stress disorder (PTSD), anxiety, or bipolar disease. I hope we can open up honest conversations so we can break down the barriers preventing good people from getting the help they need and deserve. Seeing colleague after colleague die led to an internal critical mass for me. The toll on our communities has likewise been devastating, yet little seems to change to confront the issue head-on and, tragically, people continue to die every day without having been able to share their struggles.

As long as I have a voice, I will speak out to honor those people still suffering in silence, and for those who passed away too soon. I took an oath in medicine to help other people. So, if I can make a difference in just one other person's life, then telling this story will have been worth it.

CHAPTER ONE

Beginning of the End

As a young child's heart rhythm faded to a stop, I walked off the hospital floor and got in my car with a plan to end my own life. For weeks, I had watched the life drain out of her due to a progressive, unforgiving cancer. Day after day, I witnessed her slow, agonizing death and the heartache of a young family. I felt helpless to stop the forces fighting against them. In my own state of depressed hopelessness, I felt my life slipping further and further away. Sitting in the car, I closed the door behind me like I was shutting a coffin. After the ignition started, with the wheels aligned like four pallbearers ushering a ceremonial procession, I rolled out of the hospital parking garage and headed toward absolution in the vehicle of a broken mind.

In the crisp late-fall air, I draped my left arm out the driver's-side window, hoping a cool breeze would revive a sensation behind the nothingness of feeling numb. Not feeling anything at all, I circled around the gun store parking lot one more time. The car headlight beams swept across the neon sign in the storefront window. The rolling tires seemed to hesitate suddenly, much as a knife once did while it hovered over a vulnerable vein. On that occasion, the knife never hit the skin, but deeper plans were in motion now.

After one more time around, I nestled the car between two painted yellow lines. For weeks, I had flirted with similar temptations in the form of car exhaust fumes and a slowly closing garage door. As the door came down, I saw the closure of a final chapter of my life, marked by graphic visualizations of a final gasp for air.

Living in this state of disconnected reality, I felt in moments like I was already gone. Often, I struggled to separate an impending deed from what had already been done.

As I reached for the door handle, I felt the weight of the preceding year in which, an inch at a time, I had forfeited ground from the person I had always wanted to be. Since the earliest days of my youth, I had aspired to be a healer, but after years of medical practice I felt overwhelmed, defeated, broken, and bullied by a profession that methodically stole my authentic core identity, until I felt like I had nothing left to give. I simply wanted to help people. Yet in the confines of how I was living and working in medicine, I couldn't even help myself.

The hinge creaked, and the car door swung open with an almost human tone, a noise not so much like a cry for help as a scream of despair. Straddling the door frame, I took a swig of vodka, and then placed my left foot on the ground. My right foot remained planted over a brown paper bag on the floor mat of the car as I mounted the courage to actually step outside.

A few paces to the store's front door took me to another point of no return, another framed entryway to an inevitable exit. My focus went to the backlit glass case, and a greater solution.

A dark depression had blanketed every aspect of my life over the preceding months. The consuming numbness revoked every ounce of joy from a previously ordinary life. I had survived periods of depression earlier in my medical career, but nothing like this. This time it went to a lower depth, a waking nightmare complicated by attempts to find a liquid solution to relieve the intensity of an indescribable pain. Day by day, I existed in a void, exacerbated by decades of deep-seated guilt and never feeling like I truly belonged.

For a few minutes, I meandered back and forth along the gun case, indecisive about the collection or the caliber, but knowing all the same what I needed as a mechanism of escape. I tapped my fingers gently across the glass display as my mind drifted off to a field and a welcome silence. I imagined walking through the eye-high stalks of an Indiana cornfield, my hand grazing the silk of each ear of corn. Lost in between the rows, I saw a narrow future converge into a pathless nothing. The falling sun dispersed longer shadows as I walked deeper into the labyrinth, until I started to fade away. With my hand now running down the length of the store case, I startled when the store clerk offered a casual greeting. His simple words extracted me from a deliberate self-delusion. As I turned toward the greeting, I saw a younger gentleman, a handful of years my junior, with a slender frame, a steely look, and a five-o'clock shadow.

"What can I do for you today?" he inquired.

"Searching for some protection," I answered sheepishly.

"I got just what you need over here."

All I knew was that I needed the pain to end. After a brief exchange, I found myself holding a 9mm handgun, feeling the metal pressed against my shaky, clammy palm. I held my finger over the trigger in an improvisational dry run, a prelude to a desired conclusion. I took out the cartridge and nodded my head subtly, projecting confidence as though this wasn't the first time in my life I had held a gun. I asked about the price of the bullets as I contemplated the next steps in a rapidly evolving plan.

"First gun?" the clerk asked.

"Yeah, first time needing one," I softly replied.

"Well, I'll leave these papers. Holler when you have a question." He walked over to grab a shotgun off the wall for an older gentleman standing patiently by the register.

In the moment, and for years to come, I felt the weight of holding that gun. Steel in hand, I looked down at the forms, read a few brief lines, and quickly realized it would take weeks of processing and holding periods before the weapon would be in my hands. I didn't feel like I had that kind of time.

Without another word, I abruptly retreated back into the rationalizations of an ailing mind. Step by shuffling step, I walked toward the door, forgetting about this plan and moving on to thoughts of another way to die. On the drive home, I saw only exit signs and monotonous stretches of highway ahead. I envisioned a swift turn of the steering wheel, my car veering off the bridge and sailing toward the embankment below. Instead, with street lights converging in the rear view behind me, I kept driving home. Upon arriving, I thought about what I could possibly say. As I lumbered into the kitchen I knew the words wouldn't matter anyway. At our dining room table, my wife and I ate dinner in defeated silence as I thought about my final goodbyes. With many things left unsaid, I pushed away from the table and ascended the stairs, out of sight.

The following morning, after a restful night's sleep, I woke up as I had on any other day. I kissed my wife on the forehead and then walked past framed memories from our life together hanging on the wall. Downstairs, I was greeted by the wagging tails of two Labrador retrievers, innocently welcoming the excitement of another day. For a few moments I lay on the cold tiles of the kitchen floor as the dogs' weight pinned me there, as though urging my body to stay a little while longer. Years before, we had rescued them from the beginnings of a desolate life, and I wished at that moment that they could have done the same for mine. Patting their heads, I told them about the new protective role they would have to play, and then took a few backward steps out of their lives.

My first steps onto the concrete garage floor felt like stepping out of a warm shower onto ceramic tile. I felt the cold and nothing more. Out of a sliver of the garage window, I saw leaves falling off a towering ash tree in the darkness. One by one, they seemingly leaped from unsurvivable heights, floating into a purgatory breeze for a few final moments of time. As I backed the car out of the driveway, leaf after leaf crashed to the ground, and I retreated into an inviting gray. The car's headlights clashed with the fog-filled darkness as a bottle sat on the passenger seat, and my right hand shifted the car forward into drive. In the welcoming haze, I drove to a secluded place and then walked into the woods with a feeling of comfort about the end of my life.

CHAPTER TWO

Growing up

As I was growing up, my father worked as an adolescent/young adult mental health therapist, a profession I knew he loved, but it also carried an immeasurable toll: the weight of living in the mental health stories of others while raising children of his own. We didn't speak about it much then, but I overheard enough. Whispered hallway phone calls about going back into the office because of an opioid overdose, a suicide attempt, or a patient experiencing a manic episode of bipolar disorder. With my bedroom door cracked open, I heard conversations about a patient surrendering a loaded gun to my father after having expressed a desire to shoot himself in the head. It was an ironic foreshadowing of a future life of mental health and addiction struggles, but at the time I was living on the outside of this world, inside my own home.

I often wondered, and worried, whether being a "mentally-ill addict" was a byproduct of being raised in a small, rural, poverty-stricken town. From a naive vantage point, I assumed those illnesses only existed among the men and women living in the tents underneath the highway overpass. I was told homelessness was a "consequence" of addiction in an elementary school DARE (Drug Abuse Resistance Education) program. Days after "graduating" from the program, I found a rust-eaten can of hypodermic needles in a tent by the railroad tracks a few dozen yards from my bedroom window. Later, I learned from textbooks that addiction can be influenced by both genetic and socioeconomic factors. Yet in my childhood, I only heard about the social ones. It wasn't until decades later, well after I left the confines of my small town, that I learned about my own family's addiction genes.

My father often took overnight on-call duty or covered weekend shifts to provide for our family. And on several occasions, I joined him on weekend trips to our regional hospital to check on his patients. We drove along the brick-paved Main Street of our small southern Indiana town, past an old baseball card store, with an out-of-commission grain elevator a few blocks off in the distance. I scurried in the hospital's back entrance with the exhilaration of a kid on an impromptu take-your-child-to-work day. As my father and I walked down the tile ramp, I grabbed hold of the wood railing not for stability, but to innocently explore the textures of a new and foreign world. I saw a scuffed piece of tile and wondered about the person who left that small bit of footprint behind. I envisioned scenes of a patient being wheeled frantically down the hall, white coats flapping, gurney wheels turning, a desperate family following feverishly behind. Decades later, my own story would seem less theatrical as I sat in a generic, tan-walled office next to a pile of medical articles; my own psychiatric admission process would begin, and a childhood imagination would meet a sobering reality.

I felt like a detective as I investigated a hole in the hallway wall the size of a fist. I worried about the person behind the imprint, wondering how they felt now. I could sense a deeper explanation was there, and if the hallway could talk, it would have many stories to tell. A curiosity overwhelmed me, and I knew I belonged in a hospital space and hoped one day I would have the opportunity to search for those elusive answers.

We descended a ramp toward a silver elevator bookended by plastic potted plants. I imagined that the greenery camouflaged a secret entrance to a world previously unknown as a swipe of my father's hospital badge granted us access to more parts of the building.

The sterile seriousness of the elevator car stirred an immediate emotional grounding in me—rubber soles on a metal floor. In this enclosed, quiet space, I forgot about the innocence of our father/son adventure. I could see a gravity in my father's eyes pulled by something on the other side of the elevator doors. As we rode up to the fourth floor, we were seemingly being transported not just forty feet above ground level, but into a different emotional plane altogether. In those seconds, he shifted into who he had to be for his patients, as though he were stepping into a suit of bulletproof armor. A telephone booth or dressing room wasn't required; he simply wore the new role in the expression on his face.

Later in my own career, I would feel as though I failed to follow his example, not knowing how to balance empathy for others with my own emotional needs. I did not realize the cumulative weight of trying to help other people until it was almost too late. In that hospital elevator, enclosed by stainless steel, I witnessed the arming of his self-preservation process as he prepared to perform a job well while protecting his family and his own sanity.

We walked out into a waiting area, where I meandered to a seat in the corner. I knew this was where we parted ways on our adventure. My father walked up to a reinforced-glass window to show his badge, and within moments a steel door unlocked and swung open. I could see into the holding-room area, where another locked door waited on the other side. The door closed slowly and almost begrudgingly behind him, revealing an inscription:

Inpatient Psychiatric Unit
Doors Locked at All Times

I knew he was seeing someone who was struggling, and that he had spent years building a relationship strong enough to support them through their sickness. My father was a helper who always did his best to make other people feel better. The words on the door still seemed foreign, though. I just assumed all of the hospital rooms were locked for the privacy of the patients.

This simple understanding was comforting. No deeper explanation was needed, so I focused on the child-accessible features in the room: a television set, couch, and upright piano. In a pretty regular routine, I turned on the TV then plodded over to the vinyl couch. An end table hosted a collection of old magazines meant to offer distractions for captive minds. The collection consisted mostly of medical magazines, but occasionally a *National Geographic* or *Sports Illustrated* would appear. On a previous visit, I noticed the mailing label on one of the magazines had our home address on it and realized that my father was bringing pieces of home into work with him.

In my youth, my imagination often ran wild, but my attention span struggled to keep up. After flipping through a few tattered magazine pages, I wandered over to the piano. I could feel the eyes of the middle-aged door attendant stalk me across the room; she probably hoped I wouldn't touch the piano. After a brief bow to the lone member of my audience, I pulled out the bench and scooted into performance position, feet dangling far above the pedals. In my mind, the notes were melodic and the transitions smooth, each key strike an outward expression of my inner self. In truth, I was a deeply un-self-aware child pianist—more nuisance than noteworthy, more clash than chord. Yet the instrument still freed what was captive inside me. Moments of exhilarating passion poured into a final crescendo worthy of a grand ovation, if only for the effort I'd put in.

With the final note, a great sense of joy reverberated through me. Playing piano allowed me to feel creative and deep and, best of all, distracted from a growing sense of internal discord. In the years to come, music I favored mirrored my emotional trajectory, through increasingly dark and ominous tones, and ultimately, in the depths of my depression, the bottle became the only way I knew how to drown out the chaotic frequencies around me.

When I looked up from the piano, the attendant shook her head, and the applause never came. After a moment of disappointment, I noticed a book of sheet music on a nearby stand. It was open to "Nocturne in B flat minor" by Frederic Chopin. All I saw was a score of complex lines, notes, and symbols. For the second time in this brief hospital visit, I was encountering an untranslated, locked-away world, one in clef form and another behind a steel hospital door. Both seemed intriguingly beautiful, as they hid something unknowable by outsiders like me. I wondered what it was like to have that knowledge, to be granted access to the rhythms and melodies of human expression. I wanted to unlock that mystery and discover the depths of a symphony hiding in plain sight.

"You know, one of our patients can play that song," the attendant whispered while peering at me through the window at her station.

"Really?" I said. "I'm sure it's beautiful to hear."

She shook her head in a kind of knowing condescension and closed the window. The music I played didn't seem to move her the same way that it moved me; I feared we were listening with different sets of ears. As time passed, I wondered whether that patient still liked to play, and whether the music he or she played fell on discerning ears. I hoped that other people heard the same beauty in the song and appreciated it for what it was meant to be.

I knew through trips like these that I wanted to help people when I grew up, just like my father. Medicine became a calling to discover deeper, richer levels of human experience and to help unlock the mysteries of the suffering that occurs on the other side of those steel doors.

More and more over time in my early youth, I realized that I felt deeply for other people and felt constantly intrigued by patterns of human behavior. But I was scrawny, introverted, and shy, and I became an easy target. The transition to elementary school was a difficult one, faced as I was with a lack of control and a constant struggle to fit in. I dreaded the early-morning sound of the bus tires gripping the road on the curve around the corner from our house. I saw the flashing red school bus sign as a call to the beginning of a torturous routine. On mornings when I couldn't bear it, I held a digital thermometer to a lamp bulb in my bedroom to feign a fever. The thermometer registered as high as 110 degrees. My mother knew I was faking it and disappointedly shook her head as I trudged out the front door. Sometimes she literally had to push me onto the bus with her loving but stern maternal hand; the driver grabbed my arm and pulled me inside, then slammed the door behind me. My head hung toward my shuffling feet as I made my way down the aisle. As I slid into a second row seat, I heard a fourth grader yell, "Why don't they feed you?" Another child would pile on, "I've seen toothpicks bigger than his arms." In a mob-like elementary hysteria, the insults hurled themselves over a half-dozen rows of schoolbus seats. Then, the weighted words landed where a seatbelt should have been, in the lap of an unsecured child.

Once at school, I would sneak into the classroom and hide behind a bookshelf in the corner, clutching a backpack tightly over my chest. When the morning bell rang, the teacher coaxed me out of my secluded space little by little. She worked to build trust by extending her hand, as though offering comfort to a wounded animal. As I slowly emerged, my toes tested the floor ahead of me, and I held a comfortable weight on my trailing leg, ready to flee. I felt like I didn't belong. The world seemed to be spinning out of control. I was labeled a "mama's boy" by teasing classmates and a child with "separation anxiety" by overbearing teachers. The truth was that I carried profound social anxiety as an awkward kid assimilating in a clique-filled community. I got barraged with insults for what my peers saw on the outside, so I squeezed the pack tight to compress everything I felt inside. Were I to open up and try to connect with the other kids, I expected the same harsh rejections.

I hid the pack under my desk, never opening it for more than a few moments at a time. In a rush, I would pull out a pencil and an eraser, and then hurriedly zipped the pack back up.

Outwardly, my behavior was peculiar, defensive, and against childhood norms, so the other students had taken note. The teasing began as whispers and unforgiving gazes. In their defense, it was odd for a kid to sit behind a bookshelf, eyes peering between the dust covers. I disrupted the normalcy of their morning routine. The Pledge of Allegiance went on as I attempted to hide yet stood out more and more with each patriotic word.

I felt a sense of judgment hanging over every move I made. Every trip to the chalkboard was marred by an internal screeching of fingernails across the insecurities of a tender mind. As time went on I learned that the fewer marks I made in the world, the fewer criticisms I was likely to receive. Over time, these moments bolstered me to strive for perfection to avoid conflict or judgment, a self-preservation tactic in an unforgiving world.

I did let small pieces of myself out as a kid, but repressed the full spectrum of my emotions within. I couldn't be hurt for the things I hid. I spent months coloring in black and white with an elbow fortress to block public view. I rushed up to the teacher's desk to turn in homework, but buried it in a pile of other classmates' work. But this behavior in itself attracted trouble. Being different was not going to be tolerated, and pretty soon the physical bullying started.

Arm punches, trips, and shoves out of the recess line became a daily occurrence. On a snowy winter morning, a pair of classmates, feigning interest in showing me their new winter boots, lured me into the coat room closet. A few seconds later, I felt a violent shove from behind and toppled into a basket of ice-covered gloves. The assailants scurried back to their assigned seats. There I sat, cold, alone, and startled, underneath a solitary coat hook. Looking up, I saw my favorite light-blue jacket swaying on the hook, moved by the force of my collision with the wall. Gathering my senses, I slumped down until my head met my knees, and soon tears followed. I had trained myself to wait until I was truly alone to cry, as this form of vulnerability would obviously attract additional flurries of ridicule.

When I lifted my head, I noticed my frayed backpack splayed open on the closet floor. Poking through the zipper was a kaleidoscope-style drawing and scattered broken crayons. I crawled on my hands and knees across the rug-draped concrete floor to pick up the remaining fragments of the artistic expression of my inner self.

Since I learned as a child that the world is full of bullies ready to judge, shame, and punish people for being different, for decades I practiced hiding the most sensitive parts of my life, which hindered my ability to open up to others about my mental health. In active depression and addiction, I lived out a self-fulfilling prophecy of seclusion, buttressed by the formative lessons of a fragile child.

In stark contrast to my school days, however, I received kindness at home; my parents sacrificed a lot so my siblings and I would have good opportunities. Each worked multiple jobs to ensure that we could explore our every interest and passion. Thanks to their sacrifice, I developed a love for tennis in middle school, and by the time I reached high school I was a fairly successful player on one of the state's top-ranked teams. My senior year I played doubles, and our team carried a one-loss record into the regional finals. After years of hard work and dedication to the sport, I had a realistic hope of playing for the state championship.

I often managed the remnants of my childhood insecurity by striving for perfection in every measurable manifestation of achievement. But I continued to hide lingering emotional struggles from being a shy, awkward, tormented kid. Though I received athletic and academic accolades, a pervasive anxiety remained. My bouts of anxiety felt like the crack of a thunderbolt, instantaneous and unexpected, with a reverberation of pins and needles that felt like the aftershocks of a hornet's sting. It made my chest feel heavy. Often I had to intentionally will myself to breathe. I would then freeze for a few seconds at a time, as though losing an innocent childhood game of tag and my mind at the same time.

By late high school I would also drink socially a few times a month with friends. My first drink was a cinnamon schnapps called Hot Damn 100, which I tried on a summer camp excursion with unspectacular results. There wasn't any lightbulb moment, no life-changing epiphany; I was just a teenager having fun with friends. It was the thing everyone was doing, or at least everyone in the friend group I wanted to include myself in. At the time, I was unaware of the dangerous relationship between anxiety and self-medicating, so I continued on an unassuming path of relying on alcohol to quell uncomfortable emotions during social situations for years to come.

On a Saturday night a few days before the regional tennis finals, I made a fateful decision when I consumed a few beers while lounging on the front porch of a friend's house. A few of us were celebrating a sectional tennis victory—an expression of the hubris of a sports-filled youth. From a wooden swing, I stared down the tree-lined street at shadows dancing underneath a nearby streetlight. Some classmates were having their own party just a few houses away.

I took a deep breath, thinking life couldn't get much better than this. All the years of 6 a.m. tennis lessons, blistering hot summer practices, and winters spent running outside to stay in peak condition were finally paying off. We sometimes practiced twice a day, early in the morning, then late in the afternoon. After the morning sessions ended, we would scurry off the courts, grab a quick bite, and head to an abandoned quarry pit for a swim. I saw all the dots connecting my hard work with the rewards of success. In this youthful naivete I had life all figured out. What could possibly go wrong?

Feeling liberated from the beer drinking, I jumped off the porch with the energy of a boy chasing his dog down a street. "Wait up! Wait up!" I called to the shadowy figures. I didn't feel like being left out, so I ran faster, grasping for any new chance for acceptance. It had only taken a few drinks for this level of courage. My stride lengthened as I picked up the pace, building to a sprint. I was about twenty yards from the group when I hit a curb and my ankle gave way. I tumbled over myself and crashed to the asphalt. Road-rash blood smeared the corner of my eye, but my senses flocked to a throbbing pain running up my left leg. I saw, flashing before my eyes, the dream of a tennis title dissipate with every agonizing pulse through my rapidly swelling ankle.

Afraid to tell my parents, I called my sister instead. She came and took me to the local emergency room where, in guilt and pain, I sat in a stark-white hospital hallway, waiting. Once in the triage area, I pulled my blood-stained shirt over my mouth and let out a deep sigh. When I looked up, my sister Amanda's hand was held out, offering a stick of gum. She was trying to keep me calm. We waited together, and when the X-ray results came in, I was reassured to hear that no bones were broken. The diagnosis was a severe ankle sprain, and the doctor's prescription was rest, ice, and time. But my next tennis match was five days away.

In the days to come, I worked painstakingly to rehabilitate my ankle with ice baths and stretches. I couldn't practice, and my teammates didn't hear the true story, because I couldn't bring myself to tell them what actually happened. My coach didn't want me to play, but I insisted that I was okay. So, I played through the pain with an air cast on, and we lost. I played as well as I could, but I knew I wasn't competing at 100 percent, which opened up a lifetime of wondering what could have been, as well as a reserve of unending regret. The internal turmoil rose in the days to come; I felt terribly guilty for squandering an opportunity to achieve at the highest level. It was only a game; I knew that. It was only high school; I knew that too. But after years of being the kid pushed down into trash cans, I wanted to prove I was worth more than what I thought other people saw in me. I wanted to prove those people wrong. Instead, I felt as though they were right all along.

I wallowed in shame for negating all the sacrifices my parents made to put me in a position to succeed. I felt like I had let down the people who believed in me, and my adolescent mind doubted that they would ever believe in me again. In the years to come, I buried the brewing turmoil deep inside and carried around the baggage of disappointing so many people, never fully processing the weight of what occurred. I didn't realize the emotional angst would fill every crack and crevice of my inner self, like water poured into a jar of sand. Over time, the heaviness wore me down and finally began to test the limits of how much I could carry on an already wounded frame.

CHAPTER THREE

Becoming a Bulldog

Inspired by my father, I headed to college with intentions to study psychology as a premedicine major. During the previous fall, I had toured college campuses with my mother on long weekend drives across the Midwest. Resting my head against the rolled-up window, gazing down the long stretches of open road ahead, the possibilities seemed endless. On each tour, my mind raced wildly about the opportunity for a fresh start. I wanted to leave old emotional baggage in the trunk and let my parents simply haul it away. I hoped it would be that simple. In the end, after all of the weekend drives and campus tours, I knew I was born to be a Butler University Bulldog. Butler felt like a home away from home from the minute I set foot on its Indianapolis campus. I was excited both for the benefits afforded by a big city, and to pursue a challenging career.

Those were some of the best years of my life. I took college seriously, studying late into the night and dedicating myself to the rigors of academic success. I worked two jobs, took on my own loans, held down a double major, and focused on my medical career path. Yet I can trace the early warning signs of addiction and depression back to this stage of my life, hampered as I was by a growing sense of insecurity, social anxiety, and the challenges of transitioning to a college world filled with obligations.

I usually spent my Friday nights volunteering at the local children's hospital. At nineteen years of age, I had finally gained access to the inner world of helping sick children. I pushed a toy cart around the hospital, delivering gifts to patients in some of the most difficult times of their lives. I saw families forced to make hospital couches their temporary homes, children walking the halls tethered to IV poles, and the resiliency of youthful hope as they battled diseases they should never have had to understand.

On one of those Friday evenings, I met a girl my age resting in an oncology ward hospital bed. When I handed her a stuffed animal, she smiled faintly out of a corner of her mouth and sighed in contemplation.

"My friends are at a sorority party right now, and here I am lying in this bed," she said with her eyes fixed on the plush bear's nose. She held the softness next to her face, and then tilted her head back onto her pillow, looking longingly out the tempered glass window.

I didn't know what I could possibly say, so I excused myself. Her mother thanked me, and I walked down the hall into another person's captive hospital life. A guilt rose in me then that I could walk out freely, back to my college life with no strings attached.

On a Thursday afternoon during sophomore year, a friend called to invite me to his fraternity house room. The home, constructed like a brick manor, boasted pristine views of the historic Hinkle Fieldhouse, yet time, and the recklessness of its young inhabitants, yielded notably less majesty on the inside. It had dark hallways, broken lights, and makeshift bunk beds lining poster-filled walls.

I lived in a house with four other guys, halfway between the hospital and the university. On that Thursday afternoon, I decided to drive over since classes were out for the day. Later in the evening the hallowed field house would host thousands of basketball fans, and my friends had started their preparations for the game a little early by drinking several beers during a post-lunch poker game. So, on arrival, I quickly caught up. At this point in my life, I only drank a few nights a month, but on those occasions I would binge. Over a few hours' time I had a handful of beers and realized that everyone around me seemed intoxicated, but

I could drink the same amount as they did and feel completely fine. The effects felt different to me, calming and soothing. I didn't feel sloppy or irrational; I felt a sense of peace. The anxiety I felt in crowds or amidst people I didn't know slowly evaporated. Whereas emotionally I had been sitting behind an elementary school bookshelf, I could be coaxed out by a beer to join my peers. I took on another persona while drinking—social, fun, and more likeable than the kid who was pushed into a box of frozen gloves. In short, I could be somebody else.

Later that evening, a friend said, "I can't even tell when you've been drinking, because you just act the same." The observation would stick with me for many years; I assumed I could always hide the effects of my drinking from other people. I tucked these thoughts away, relying on them to solidify a belief that would support my future secret life. And I felt validated that I could keep this secret.

In truth, I didn't stop drinking the way other people stopped. I would often drink longer than anyone else at a party, not noticing that friends had some internal barometer for knowing when enough was enough. Once I started, I accelerated past off-ramps of moderation time and time again, because I always felt like having one more.

A year later, on a deserted stretch of highway, I witnessed the collateral damage of navigating life with the pedal carelessly pressed to the floor. I was home for summer vacation and my father and I had driven to St. Louis to see a Cardinals game on a humid Friday night. A little after 10 p.m., after the game ended in a hometown victory, we strolled back to the car for the drive home. I took the wheel for the three-hour drive, and we talked about life and baseball, but mostly about baseball. No matter the conversation, how casual or how professional, my father always found a way to bring it back to the game he loved. Even when I excitedly announced my decision to attend Butler, he had said, "That's great, son. Cardinals are up 7–4 in the eighth inning."

My father had had a few beers during the game, but I had abstained, knowing I would drive home. In my entire life, I've only seen my father intoxicated once. He was always measured and precise in his drinking, having one or two beers, no more. There was a reason behind his measured approach. It stemmed from the heartache of a lived experience, as his grandfather's consumption had been a different story altogether. My great-grandfather passed away from a failing heart due to alcoholism. My grandfather Bob and my father Mark both lived with the burden of seeing the catastrophic demise of a man in the prime of his life. They both lived with the knowledge that a spiral of addiction was only one family member removed from them, and they took fewer chances because of it.

A love of baseball is a bit of a Hill family tradition, so I thought about my father's side of the family as we left the Gateway Arch and the lights of the city behind. We cruised in the left lane behind a convoy of semi trucks and passed the sprawling suburban outlet exits, comfortably on our way home.

My father asked, "How about that double play at the top of the second inning?" But just as I started to reply, I saw something out of the corner of my eye and screamed, "Oh my God!"

A vehicle had drifted across two lanes of speeding traffic; the flow of eastbound traffic was suddenly confronted by a northbound vehicle. The collision was abrupt and violent, and I felt the pavement shake beneath us. The high-impact domino cascade started a single car length ahead, and I sensed the approach of the truck convoy that was now behind us.

The next moments froze into singular segments of time. We crashed at full speed into the car in front of us as the pileup consumed several vehicles traveling in the next lane. The air bags deployed with a blast of white powder and the smell of an ignited chemical burn. Each second was an actionable moment to fight for survival. In a move of blind faith, with a single turn of the wheel, we managed to avoid being further enveloped in the ongoing mayhem. On two flat tires, and with a startled consciousness, I drove until we were a few hundred yards from the wreckage.

As our car stopped, I looked out the shattered front window to see the hood folded like an accordion. Through the back window I saw masses of crumpled metal, with headlights illuminating cornfields instead of the road's yellow lines. The lights of one of the vehicles, now lying on its hood, pointed upward into the dark Illinois sky.

Acting on instinct, my father and I both jumped out of the car, grabbed a first-aid kit and flashlight from the trunk, and ran back toward the scene. As I ran, the flashlight beam bounced off the pavement like a luminescent ping-pong ball. I feared what I would see upon arrival, accepting the near certainty that I would never unsee it. I rushed toward the inciting car, which was smashed into the median guardrail. As I approached, I heard the screams of a young girl, her voice carrying across the empty highway ahead. Inside the tortured steel, a teenage boy was slumped over the steering wheel, blood dripping down his forehead, and his sister, battered and shaken, was at his side. The door of the car was gone, so I leaned my head through the space where the window had been. I smelled alcohol in the car and then again on the driver's breath. I watched his breathing patterns, taking some comfort in seeing the consistent rise and fall of his chest. We helped them out, and tried to assess what had caused the gruesome scene.

Once they were out of the road, I covered them in blankets, and we sat on the side of the highway waiting for first responders to arrive. Off in the distance, a host of flashing blue and red lights finally appeared. I looked back toward the wreckage in utter disbelief that everyone had survived the incredible destruction. I sensed the immense amount of collateral damage—thousands of lives altered in the wake of a boy's fateful decision. With an arm draped around a young stranger, I thought about the split-second decisions I had made that prevented someone else's alcohol use from taking my life. At the time, I thought I knew which side of the wreckage I would never be on.

A year later, when memories of the accident had faded into the background, I began preparing for the Medical College Admission Test (MCAT), the entrance exam for medical school. That semester, one of the courses I took in the pharmacy department was "The History of

Drug Culture." I was fascinated by subcultures surrounding drug use and figured the course might be useful in my future career. We learned the origin stories of countercultures and how medications and drugs of abuse had evolved throughout history, from the Harrison Act, which taxed and regulated opiates, to the formation of the Drug Enforcement Administration (DEA), to the Durham-Humphrey Amendment which defined prescription and over-the-counter medications, to Ronald Reagan's "War on Drugs." All of it captivated me, and, to be honest, it still does to this day. One of the most striking parts of the course came toward the end of the semester, when our professor brought a panel of six individuals into our classroom. They each had active, untreated substance use conditions or were in varying stages of recovery.

Our professor introduced the first panel member as a local pharmacist, then calmly handed the microphone to the scruffy, middle-aged man. He was slight of build and had slumped shoulders. "Well, my name is Reggie and I lost everything because I'm a drug addict," he said.

A hush fell over the room, the kind of silence where a pipe creak can seem deafening. My bottom lip fell half an inch and I became conscious of every breath I took.

Reggie went on: "I wouldn't even know where to start, but I guess I just always felt different and uncomfortable in my own skin."

In the twenty minutes that followed, he spoke of losing everything in his life and career. He shared about the first time he took a prescription bottle from his parents' bedroom, and about using his work to access more pills. He relied on painkillers to live up to their name, and the pills delivered on that promise in a Faustian bargain that almost cost him his life—twice. The second time, he was carried out of his home on a stretcher and into an ambulance. According to his hazy recollection, he remembered waking up the next day in an intensive care unit with no family or friends left to greet him—no flowers, no balloons, and no one who could endure the collateral carnage of his battle any longer. Over the course of only a few years, his addiction cost him his job, wife, house, and children. Not long afterward, he found himself scouring dumpsters for pieces of scrap metal to sell to enable his next euphoric dance with heroin. He talked about being in recovery for several years, and revealed that the feelings of longing never left him. He struggled daily to fill the void.

"I never was able to regain what I once had," he said.

I was not really sure whether he was referring to the longing for another use of the needle or for his family, his house, and his former job. I feared it was not the latter.

Reggie said, "I only felt like me when I was using."

These words triggered an immediate flashback to the fraternity house a few months earlier where, as alcohol coursed through my body, a warmth poured over me, like slowly melting into a bathtub at the end of an exhausting day.

I absorbed everything he said, hanging closely onto every unpleasant word. His mesmerizing tale unearthed in me a strangely misplaced affection. I did not pity him, nor did I judge him; I understood exactly what he was trying to express. The way he talked, the way he moved, and the way he romanticized his life shook me to the core. I focused on his description of the release he felt from all the struggles in his life when the needle hit his arm, more so than on the grimy alley where the needle was found. I wanted to hear more about his using, rather than descriptions of his kids. And I wanted to know why someone I had never met knew me better than anyone else in my life.

The words he chose to paint a picture of a calmer sense of being struck me: Release. Relief. Warmth. Numb.

I had very little experience with recreational drugs at the time, and was not conscious yet of my using them for self-medication; but it still made sense to me. I understood a perpetual cycle of filling a void with fleeting moment of peace and relief. I related to finally feeling comfortable in one's own skin, in taking a chemical path to breathe deeply and calmly, and to quieting the chaos if only for a moment.

That day, I met my own addiction before my addiction met me. Then, as young people tend to, I buried the thought and moved on to the next thing.

I really loved the class and my entire experience at Butler University, a place that to this day I find to be a home away from home. Butler taught me "The Butler Way" of humility, commitment, unity, servanthood, and teamwork, and with this foundation I felt prepared for the next steps of professional success.

With this preparation, toward the end of my time as a undergraduate, I applied to medical schools all over the country. I was an average candidate because of a borderline score on the MCAT. I will admit I have never been a great standardized test taker. Even with a 3.75 grade-point average, a double major with lots of extracurricular activities, and a solid resume, I was lumped into the category of "a risk" because of my low test scores. These categorizations were meant to predict future success. And so, because of those academic algorithms, for the first time in my life I was labeled a risk.

After applying to twenty schools, I heard back from only three. And of the three, I was offered two interviews, one being with the medical school in my home state, Indiana University. I was excited to get the formal interview, knowing that if I could just get a foot in the door, I would have a chance. But the interviews came and went, and I waited.

And I waited.

Eventually, after a few months, I received one letter in the mail, a wait-list letter.

Apparently I wouldn't be worthy of a spot unless more-qualified applicants declined. I had no idea how far down on the backups list I was, so I waited as several months rolled by. In late April, I approached graduation with a daunting uncertainty about my future. I had studied to be a doctor and nothing less. I had no backup plan.

After graduation, I waited tables at an Italian restaurant on the north side of the city as I waited to hear. My lifelong dream seemed to be fading as I closed down the restaurant night after night. After closing at 1 a.m. a couple servers would sit at the bar, have a few drinks, and complain about the poor tips, angry patrons, and annoying high school students who tried to order alcohol with fake IDs. We laughed, we drank, and I worried. I drove home from each shift questioning every decision I had ever made in my life, wondering if I was good enough, or if I should have done more. The sense of inferiority had surfaced once again.

This went on for a few weeks. I would get home a little after 2 a.m., sleep into the late morning, and stalk the mail carrier in the afternoon, waiting for the mail to arrive. Six weeks went by like this without a word, as whispered self-abasements rose continually from the darkest depths of my mind.

You didn't do enough.

You don't deserve this opportunity.

I hated myself for hating myself, but I didn't have the power to stop. As I kept repeating the mantras of self-deprecation, I grudgingly forced myself out to the car each afternoon for another shift. In these weeks, I felt the first inklings of a brewing depression—but it was temporarily relieved by a moment soon to come.

One day on the drive to work I received a call from my roommate Kevin.

"There's a big envelope in the mailbox. It looks like an official one and it's from Indiana University. What do you want me to do?"

"Open it!" I exclaimed.

Terrified and excited, I felt a full spectrum of emotions in anticipation of hearing the letter's contents. Kevin started reading, and before long I found myself pulled over on the side of the road, crying with my head in my hands.

Kevin read, "It is our great pleasure to inform you . . ."

The sweetest words I could have ever imagined—I got in.

Chapter Four

A Medical Education

"This guy sure didn't miss any meals," a classmate said, pointing at a cadaver.

I paused for a moment, struck by the insensitivity of what was happening around me. *This is not normal behavior*, I thought to myself.

Moments later, a little after 8 p.m. on a weeknight, I sat outside the anatomy lab eating a ham and cheese sandwich, acutely aware that 90 percent of taste is smell. When the five-minute break ended, I headed back into the lab to finish the evening cram session, cynically thinking that the aroma of formaldehyde may help ease my digestion. I walked toward a stepstool as the thick air, saturated with chemicals, awaited an impending desecration.

I put one foot up on the metal-alloy table as a colleague handed me the necessary tools. I lifted the other foot and planted it so that now I was straddling the remains of a human body. Only a few feet off of the ground, I wasn't prepared for the rarefied air I was about to breathe in.

A blunt wooden handle supported a row of hacksaw teeth dulled from so many students cutting into deceased human beings. Using a hacksaw on another person felt like a crime against humanity. Yet I had instructions to follow, an assignment to complete, and it was necessary to dissociate emotionally from the task at hand. As students, we weren't told the cadaver's real name, so we named him Oliver. Giving him a name felt like the only human thing we could do. His hair was still long in the back but balding on the top. He seemed to have only lived into his early 60's, and from the anchor and chain tattoo on his shoulder, I assumed his years of Navy service. All I knew of Oliver was sacrifice, from his ink mark symbol of service to his bodily gift to our medical classroom. So, I thanked him, and then I sawed into Oliver's skull. Cut after cut, I embarked on a sensitive emotional voyage with only a crude set of tools in hand.

A few weeks later, our first exam scores were posted. On that single piece of paper, I saw a flurry of red-inked insults against everything I once thought I knew. In medical school, the top academic students are skimmed from the bell curve and redistributed across a new curve without any consideration for the psychological impact this has on their fellow students' self-worth.

Now, I had seemingly fallen from being one of the top students in my entire school to one of the dumbest in my classroom. Overnight, validations of 98 percent turned into an insulting 63 percent. Smiley-face stickers morphed into slash marks and inner monologues on how I should do better.

I wondered, *If I am no longer excelling as a student, who am I?*

I struggled with this intellectual leveling, in a feeling of metaphorical thuds down the ladder of academic achievement. I felt the reality of having to readjust to underachievement, when academic success had been one of the core aspects of my identity. Since early childhood, I learned to mask feelings of physical and emotional insecurity through high academic achievement. In the medical school leveling, the mask was stripped away, and I felt exposed as a failure, an imposter, and as someone unworthy of the opportunity before him.

To compensate, I studied harder and longer, burning the candle at both ends, since medical schools recruit and reward perfectionist personalities. Pushing myself more and more, I pulled all-night study sessions, staying up thirty or more hours and then taking tests. I didn't drink often during those initial medical school years, as I simply didn't have the time. I studied, occasionally ate, slept when I could, and lost ten pounds from an already slender frame. The cycles of night and day blurred into a recognition of only artificial versus natural light shining on the words of a turning textbook page. Superstitiously, I only ate certain meals before tests and always wore the same undershirt for anatomy reviews. I shaved my head as if that would remove barriers preventing the words in the physiology book from getting into my head. I calculated that less hair somehow meant more intellectual osmosis.

The grind became exhausting, and after a year I began to feel its cumulative effect. I no longer wanted to get out of bed in the morning, I struggled to care about the events of the day, and I started to isolate myself from family and friends. I went to class, studied, and slept, then repeated that cycle again and again.

I knew something was physically wrong, so I visited the campus health office to see a doctor. A unique thing that happens to medical students over the course of their studies; they develop a hypochondria-like condition in which they experience the symptoms of illnesses they study. In the abnormality of intense hours of endless studying, I read about one abberant bodily malfunction after another, and finally started to feel the diseases lying within me. Once I felt the symptoms, the shock waves of anxiety returned, heightening the perception of danger of a rapidly progressive disease. This is referred to as medical student syndrome, or second-year syndrome, when every isolated twitch of your body is the acute onset of amyotrophic lateral sclerosis (ALS), commonly referred to as Lou Gehrig's disease, and every cough must be the end stages of a progressive lung cancer. Putting this philosophy into practice, I went into the campus health center saying, "I think I am hypothyroid. I need to have my TSH checked." Abnormal thyroid-stimulating hormone (TSH) levels could have explained the fact that I had no energy and felt like sleeping all the time. High TSH levels might have also explained my loss of appetite and lack of focus. But my levels were normal.

At the time, I had no conscious awareness that I was actually experiencing symptoms of clinical depression; I simply checked the hypothyroid diagnosis off the list and went on my way. I could not wait to see what the next day would bring—maybe Raynaud's disease or systemic lupus erythematosus.

At the beginning of my third year of medical school I started on clinical rotations, routinely seeing patients for the first time in my career. The first rotation was a six-week assignment in a surgical intensive care unit. Medical students were required to arrive by 4:30 a.m. to gather all the overnight information on the patients from the medical charts and the bedside nurses. Then the clinical rounds with the surgery residents took place a little before 6 a.m. Usually, this just meant waking patients up from deep slumbers, which pissed them off something fierce, and then running off to the operating room by 7 a.m. There, sometimes for twelve hours at a time, I would stand and watch, mindful not to make any sudden movements, talk louder than a whisper, or touch anything at all. I knew what happened with any deviation from this protocol; rumors circulated that a few months earlier a medical student had been kicked out of the OR and made to stand in the hallway for the final three hours of a complex bowel-perforation surgery. So, I just stood in silence, imagining the joy of a restroom break or a nice sit-down meal at the hospital café. This schedule did not deviate, six days a week. I would get home at around 9 p.m., shower, maybe eat, collapse, and dread the 3:45 a.m. alarm clock ring. The hours were long, the sleep was short. And social encounters (at least those that weren't dreams) were minimal, brief, and filled with the inevitable frustration of a patient whose sleep I interrupted.

One of our adult patients was in a prolonged coma after an unsuccessful attempt to remove a cancerous obstruction from his lower intestine. He was on a ventilator machine, and his body wore all the bruises of an extended fight. He was in his late forties, had a young family, had everything to lose, and was actively losing it all. A few days after his surgery, one of the resident surgeons asked our group of medical students if we wanted to practice blood draw arterial sticks on him. I sat shocked by the offer, and the casual nature of the replies. Chipper classmates sounded eager to check the procedure off their lists of technically achievable goals. Seeing this all as highly unethical, I protested.

"You can't just poke around on someone for no good reason." The words I forced out sounded like a nagging country music song.

"He can't feel it anyway," I heard someone say as I turned to walk away.

It was a moment where hypocrisy and Hippocrates collided. I hoped the other students didn't take up the offer. I never found out if they did, though, and I never asked.

There are memories we all hold firmly, sometimes without fully understanding why. I can vividly recall being in the shower at 9 p.m. with my head hanging down, not knowing how I could wake up and do it all over again. I remember this moment like it was yesterday; it's a memory I once wished I could forget. I did not realize the image of the hanging head in the shower had nothing at all to do with being on a surgery rotation; it was a foreshadowing of the brokenness I would feel in the years to come.

A few months later, I spent time working in an inpatient child psychiatric hospital, in what became my first exposure to patients with mental health stories of their own. Here, I saw signs of abuse and neglect, of children kept in dog cages, burned with cigarettes, and beaten to within an inch of their lives. These are moments the mind cannot unsee or unhear, and they are difficult to decompress from. I struggled with anger and sadness from the gut-wrenching cruelty I was exposed to. In my own emotional maturation process, I was not ready to accept these realities, and they haunted me for years. I did not know how to escape the fraught image of a child tied to a bed or sexually assaulted by their own parent. I had no concept of how to unpack the unspeakable weight of bearing witness to this level of suffering. None of my colleagues spoke about the gravity of it; for me the trauma meant an extra layer of stress on an already weary mind.

My most fulfilling experiences were working in the pediatric intensive care unit and on the pediatric oncology and stem cell transplant floors doing difficult but meaningful and impactful work. During those rotations, I grew close to a patient—a little girl named Zoe—and her family.

Zoe was a two-year-old living with a rare autoimmune condition associated with frequent life-threatening infections, and her only chance for long-term survival was to receive a stem cell transplant. Zoe was beautifully shy, an inquisitive toddler with piercing blue eyes and an illuminating smile. She loved Thomas the Train and watching early-afternoon cartoons.

I met Zoe and her family after her stem cell transplant. Over the course of her months in the hospital we formed an intimate bond. I would go visit her after rounds and we would lie on her hospital bed and watch TV or play with her trains. Over time, her sterile, quarantined room felt more like a toddler's playroom, a testament to her indomitable spirit. I marveled at her persistent ability to remain a kid while living through so much hour by hour. The resolute nature of her innocence was truly something to witness. Years later, her mother told me I had helped to maintain a bit of normalcy amidst the medical chaos unfolding before their eyes, though at the time I didn't know that was humanly possible.

Tragically, a few months later, Zoe died from complications of her transplant. I was out of town, working at another hospital, and felt ashamed that I could not be there for her in those final days or even say goodbye. Hers was the first funeral I ever attended for a child, with flower wreaths over a three-foot casket. Surrounding the receiving line were photographs of Zoe in her Easter dress and ponytail in a backyard swing. With tearful eyes, I imagined her family picking those photos off her bedroom dresser to post them on a sterile funeral-parlor wall.

Zoe was the beginning for me—she brought out who I wanted to be in medicine. She became my first true mentor, showing me what it meant to show up, how to vulnerably expose a heart to a patient, and how to care for them as a person first.

I loved that little girl, and I still do.

Years later, during our second pregnancy, my wife and I received our eighteen-week ultrasound report. I messaged Zoe's mother to ask for her blessing, as we had a name picked out: Zoe Grace.

After the funeral, I said my goodbyes and went straight to a basketball court—ninety-four feet of Indiana therapy, I suppose. It was the final game of a summer recreational league, and at the beginning of the second half I came down with a rebound and another player fell underneath me. I felt a crunch and an unnatural sensation of bone grinding against bone. I fell straight to the floor, writhing in pain, with the excruciating sensation of a piece of me tangibly breaking. A few teammates helped me off the floor and a friend took me to the hospital.

An MRI confirmed the tibial plateau fracture. No surgery required, only one day allowed off from medical school, and for eight weeks I would have to use crutches. In constant pain, I returned to work at an outpatient neurology office, after which I spent a month at a family practice. Working day after day with a braced, immobile leg for the full eight weeks, the physical injury, and the temporary loss of independence, pushed my wounded psyche over the edge.

I smiled through the day, but the internal turmoil kept rising. I had spent years hiding my vulnerability, ashamed of standing out from the crowd and afraid of what people would say or how I might be judged. But now I couldn't hide the limping any longer; I felt broken, helpless, and exposed. The physical injury became a convenient excuse for the brokenness I had carried for years. It felt okay to not feel okay, when everyone could see and understand the pain I felt from the fracture. It became clear to me for the first time, then, that I was depressed. My family helped me find a psychiatrist and counseling group and I started taking an antidepressant. At the time I did not even think twice about it. My family saw I needed help, so I accepted the help. I just wanted to feel better.

The next eight weeks were difficult, but my mood seemed to stabilize over the course of the following rotations. Honestly, one of the hardest parts was being on two outpatient electives and having to see twenty-five or more patients per day. It was not the workload or even navigating the narrow halls on crutches that proved difficult; it was that every single time I walked into a patient's room, they would ask, "What happened to *you?*" I grew to hate the unwanted sympathy. I did not want to be pitied; I just wanted to be left alone. Comically, my sister made me a T-shirt after I told her about the barrage of questions from colleagues and patients. It had block letters stating, "Yes, it is broken. I did it playing basketball. Yes, it hurts. I will still be a good doctor."

I loved that T-shirt, but truth be told, I really wanted one that said, "Yes, I am broken. It happened during medical school. It really hurts. I do not feel like a good person."

With family support, the antidepressant, and counseling, I finished the final year of medical school in a better emotional space and readied for the next step in my young career, a residency in pediatrics in St. Louis, Missouri. After a year of doing well, I decided with my doctor to discontinue the antidepressant, believing that a lot of the triggering events were due to the broken leg and the strains of medical school.

But hindsight is not always 20/20.

Chapter Five

Taking Up Residency

Sometime early in my pediatrics residency the symptoms of depression crept back into my life, so I sought counseling and restarted an antidepressant. The depression felt like being covered in the drowning density of a blanket under water, heavy and downward bound. On the best days, I'd tread water with an enveloping weight, and on the worst I felt my head sink for several minutes at a time. For the first time ever, I sought colleagues' opinions on whether treatment would affect my future job prospects. The common perception in the medical field is that seeking any form of mental health treatment or counseling will drastically diminish the opportunities in your career. There is some truth to that perception, and I would learn it the hard way in the years to come. Some friends counseled me against treatment, while others remained cautiously skeptical that it would impact my career. Ultimately, since treatment had worked for me in the past, I was willing to try it again. I truly needed it, and was naive then to what I know now about the professional consequences.

I met my future wife, Lauren, during this period, and she stood by me during the difficult times. Lauren was a St. Louis native. She graduated from St. Louis University and then landed a job working as a clinical research coordinator for a prestigious orthopedics program at Washington University. We met online, years before that was socially acceptable, and went to a St. Louis Cardinals game on our first date. When I showed up at her door, she answered wearing a baseball glove. Although she expected to, she didn't actually catch a foul ball at the game, but I found her ambition immediately endearing. Lauren is a strikingly beautiful woman, on the inside and out, with blonde hair, blue eyes, and a benevolent heart—a heart that saved my life when I needed it most.

For those three years of residency, she supported me and our two Labrador rescue puppies so I could continue to chase my professional dreams. However, I ground through the experience with the mentality of surviving year by year, believing: *Everything will be better next year, I can put my own happiness on the back burner . . . Once I am a senior resident life will be easier, I just have to keep pushing my way through . . . When I become a fellow work will be so much more fulfilling . . . Maybe when I am a faculty physician I will be happy ever after.*

Unfortunately, that optimism did not last forever, and the tactic of delaying my own pursuit of happiness came back to haunt me in the years to come.

Concurrently with this tactic, I delayed the emotional processing of tragic human events, such as one on Christmas Day of my second year of pediatric residency. I was sitting by myself in the call room at 9 p.m., after evening rounds. An eighteen-inch Christmas tree sat on the windowsill while snow fell past the tempered glass. All I had were white walls, one computer desk, and a scented candle that had been smuggled in, as open flames were against hospital policy. We never lit the candle; it was more of a rebellious gesture, and the smell was comforting. On that night, it reminded me of how much I missed being home for the holidays.

I sat alone, sorry to spend Christmas away from my family and friends for the first time. I had worked halfway through a thirty-hour call shift when my pager went off with back-to-back messages—two digital alerts to impending crises. The first page originated in the oncology unit, and the other came from the emergency room. I rushed off to the oncology floor to find a six-year-old patient having a prolonged seizure. We administered medications but were unable to stabilize him, so the intensive care team rushed in and he was urgently transferred off the floor. The boy was placed on a ventilator, and a short time later a CT scan found a significant blood clot in his brain.

No time to reflect; I was already running down the back stairwell to the emergency department. A six-month-old baby with a complex heart condition was being evaluated for increased work in breathing, decreased oxygen saturations, and an elevated heart rate. Within minutes, the monitor rhythms faded, then slowed to a stop. There I was, on Christmas evening, doing chest compressions on a six-month-old infant while a family emotionally melted into the crevices between the tiles of the waiting room floor. I performed chest compressions on the baby for thirty-five minutes, restoring no rhythm and no pulse and feeling as though nothing I could possibly say or do would comfort a family losing their infant child.

Three more pages came. I was expected to walk up the back stairwell to admit three more children to the hospital and pretend that nothing else had happened.

I did not talk about what I had just lost, because it paled in comparison to what others were actively losing. I felt ungrateful for questioning my own feelings when a family had lost their child and another child was critically ill in the intensive care unit. I was trained to function in a way that acknowledged that my needs mattered less than the needs of other people. When those personal needs are emotional ones, and we are continuously told not to pay attention to them, not to talk about them, and not to get too affected in front of patients, well, depression can feel just like another bodily function that must be suppressed. So, I went back to my call room and collapsed in the corner of the room with my knees to my chest, rocking and shaking to the bone. I looked over at the unlit candle, desperately wishing a simple match could combat the enclosing darkness. For a brief moment I started to reflect on my feelings, but then another set of beeps demanded attention. This time the page was from the oncology faculty physician wanting an update on the patient who had been transferred to the ICU—an abrupt insistence to stop feeling, stop processing, and to start the next task. As I stared past the mini Christmas tree in the window, I remembered that I had three more patients who were waiting for beds, and one family was angry because they had waited in the emergency room all day long.

Their anger began to stir up feelings about all the things that had gone wrong in my years of practicing medicine. Instead of reflecting upon the events of the present moment, I was flooded with guilt about events that happened years before, and the shame started to consume me. At one point earlier on in my career I was on a medical team that accidentally dosed a patient with a potent antibiotic that was ten times the appropriate level, causing an injury to the patient. The antibiotic damaged their kidneys, and the patient spent weeks recovering on a dialysis machine. The patient did eventually recover, the events were disclosed to the family, processes were followed, and appropriate steps taken; but us medical professionals never discussed it. We were never given a space to process our guilt, worries, and fears. In truth, we felt sick about it, and most of us still do. But we were actively discouraged from talking about it at all due to the risk of legal culpability. We all knew that once lawyers get involved, "anything you say can and will be used against you."

In early January, a few weeks later, I sat down with a mother at the bedside of her critically ill child. Her eight-year-old daughter was born with a severe brain malformation and was admitted to the hospital for an increased frequency of seizures and difficulty tolerating the nutrition in her feeding tube. The mother was sobbing at the girl's bedside, recounting all the hopes she had for her daughter when she was born. She had painted the bedroom walls bright pink and filled her daughter's room with fairy-tale figurines, teddy bears, and a whole shelf of books. She lamented how, over time, the teddy bears disappeared, the books went unread, and the fairy tale characters slowly found their way into storage to make room for feeding tubes, medications, and suction machines. Piece by piece, a mother's dreams for her daughter had been consigned to a closet while the child's bedroom turned into a triage space.

Walking out of that room, I carried the weight of all the patients previously under my care. I was heartbroken for this young mother seeing her daughter slowly fade away due to the progressive nature of her disease. A synapse was triggered in my head, taking me back to the experience of losing a child with a similar condition years before. In the grief of that memory, others flooded in, such as when four children died on the same floor of the hospital over a two-week period. One of those kids was an otherwise healthy three-year-old girl who choked on a hot dog during an ordinary afternoon meal. In her hospital bed, her headful of tiny brown curls were twirled around the wires of the EEG leads. The way she was loved sparkled in the artificial light, as a toe-sized oximeter hovered over her tiny pink nails. It was summer, and her skin still wore the suntan lines of a backyard pool in July. She should have been resting on a sun-drenched summer towel—or anywhere else but there.

I spent several intimate weeks with that family in the ICU as they tried to process the devastating, inexplicable tragedy. Their tears set the somber scene as they watched over their daughter in an ICU bed and I sat on the hospital floor having a tea party with her preschool-aged siblings.

After the final imaginary tea cups were poured, I left the building, went back to my apartment, and poured a real drink. After several months of witnessing heartache, pain, and loss, I needed a reprieve. In the same pattern as in high school and college, I didn't drink often while working six days a week and thirty-hour shifts, but when I did, I made it count. A single drink turned into a half dozen as I stared at the walls of my basement apartment, trying to grasp the depth of an entire family's loss. I replayed those innocent conversations with the five-year-old as she tried to pour tea for her baby sister on a life-support machine. When her sister didn't respond, she simply rested the cup on the bedside table. As I thought about our time together, I got drunk, and eventually I fell asleep on the living room couch with my scrubs still on.

To this day, if I go to a summer barbecue, I think of that little girl. Hot dogs over an open flame overwhelm and return my senses to the mood not of casual outdoor fun, but of a dark hospital room and a dying child. For my own children, I chop a hot dog into a million pieces before letting them eat it—each cut being a lifesaving measure in my mind. Similarly, when I walk by a pool or lake with my children, my anxiety builds as I think of the nine children I have taken care of who drowned. Power lines remind me of a teenager who was electrocuted, aspirin of a patient's deadly overdose, and the roaring of a lawnmower of a violent, ghastly scene that I can't even begin to describe for you. Medical professionals never forget these moments. We are human in our experiences, and the memories remain close to the surface and can be suddenly triggered by the mundane encounters of everyday life. Sometimes thinking about them woke me up in the middle of the night, and sometimes it prevented me from falling asleep at all.

On that night, assisted by alcohol, I remained asleep on the couch until I heard the alarm clock ring in the other room at 6 a.m. I felt glum, weary, and hung over. But there was no time for rest; the day promised another thirty-hour shift, and more opportunities to bury complex emotions deep down inside.

After morning patient rounds, I went back to the call room bathroom and splashed handfuls of cold water on my face. I looked in the mirror and saw only a silhouette of exhaustion. Before I could sit down I heard a knock at the door, and I lumbered over to answer.

"Dr. Hill, I brought you something," a friendly nurse said. It was an IV starter kit and a bag of saline. She offered the same casual nod as my sister once did while sitting in the emergency room with her injured baby brother. Behind closed doors, secretly setting up intravenous fluids for a doctor, the nurse added, "I hope this helps you get through the day."

On that particular day, a bag of fluids rejuvenated me, but the relief was temporary. It took years to process these events, even with antidepressant medication and counseling. I did not speak of the fear, anxiety, dread, or relentless foreboding about my inability to handle the trauma I witnessed every single day. I did not know I needed to, and the expectation was that no one would ever speak about it at all.

I share these stories because the events we witness in medicine are not normal; in fact, they are exceptionally abnormal. I performed CPR on a dying child without even a minute to process the event, and then it was on to the next emergency. I sat in the presence of a mother's heartache for her daughter's broken dreams, and I witnessed a team accidentally injure a patient, without so much as a moment to reflect on the emotional toll. I watched a healthy child die from an unexplainable tragedy without processing the profound human cost. Over and over, I absorbed tragedies while forcefully burying the emotional trauma deep inside in order to conform to a set of onerous standards that continue to dehumanize us all.

Before graduating from my residency, and with several more years' worth of emotional baggage weighing me down, I went off the antidepressants again.

In retrospect, that decision almost cost me my life.

Chapter Six

Dark Days

After I completed my residency, Lauren and I moved halfway across the country, leaving family and friends behind, so that I could continue my training in pediatric hematology and oncology in North Carolina. Three weeks before moving, we got married, but there was no time for a honeymoon; we simply packed up and moved on to the next stage of training and life.

We were excited and ready to take on a new adventure in our lives, so we rented a house in a sprawling residential area of Durham called Hope Valley Farms. Even though we were well below the Mason-Dixon Line, there was nary a Southern accent to be heard in our tidy neighborhood.

The Raleigh/Durham/Chapel Hill area is often referred to as the Research Triangle, and the neighborhood was filled with transplants like us: young professional couples from all over the country, juggling careers in healthcare or high tech while starting families and lives together. We loved the people, the area, the universities, and the opportunity to explore a new life together as a newlywed couple.

I knew the work would be difficult, but I felt intellectually prepared to enter into a challenging career. Most people hear about pediatric cancer as a career choice and have a visceral reaction. Whenever flying on an airplane or being introduced to someone new socially, I would simply say "pediatrician" instead of "pediatric oncologist," because the reaction was always the same—"Oh, that is such sad job"—and I cringed at the insinuation of pity. Hearing that, I would recall limping down the narrow hallways of an outpatient clinic on crutches, and I grew tired of the same, worn-out reactions. In my mind, pity meant weakness, which grated on my vulnerable psyche. Often I found myself in postures of defensive justification, and it all felt so rehearsed and inauthentic. It felt like a constant litmus test, in that I had to accept their pity, then explain the meaningfulness of my daily work; and if I failed to do so sincerely enough, they would certainly think I didn't really love my job at all.

I have always felt comfortable working with sick children and their families. However, I was not prepared for everything else that would come with the privilege of working in modern medicine. I was still operating in a mind-set of just getting through the worst parts, using a back-burner strategy to delay any greater sense of gratification, and burying complex emotions. And I was still hoping I could practice an idealized version of medicine, with autonomy, in a personally meaningful way.

I took for granted how well supported I had been in residency, when family and friends were close by, and I had not anticipated what would fill the void in their absence. I came into my fellowship with a new sense of accomplishment, and as a result, I set higher personal expectations. I had hoped the fellowship would provide more opportunities to spend time with patients and their families, but instead I was scheduling appointments, while filling out endless binders of menial paperwork. As I sat behind piles of papers, childhood memories flooded back—memories of being invited onto the recess playground, only to be tripped into a puddle of mud.

Over time, I realized that I spent more time in front of computer screens than with patients. This started out as a nuisance, built to a frustration, and then became a burdensome reality. For a decade I had studied hard to learn deductive reasoning—to identify a problem and then implement a solution. I spent sleepless night after sleepless night learning complex medical analytics designed to make a difference in people's lives.

Yet for every problem I uncovered, hours of being on the phone with an insurance company to seek approval for the treatment plan awaited. On the phone, I was often called a "provider" and asked what the "consumer" was requesting, a transactional, cash-register reduction of complex medical considerations about a patient's life. When the phone call ended with an inevitable insurance rejection, I then had to absorb the anger of the family, while feeling powerless to change any of it at all. In the interest of self-preservation, I started to feel less and less willing to walk into a room with yet another patient. I realized that only more problems awaited there, and I lacked tangible solutions. In the manner of a conflict-avoidant child, I learned to protect myself by minimizing the ability of other people to cause me harm. Over a short amount of time, I grew angry and resentful at what my daily life had become. On the outside I could stand in composed silence, while under the surface things were building to a boil. I saw the passion I had for helping other people eroded by a stifling bureaucracy, and pushed aside in favor of endless forms and templates to fill in and computer boxes to click.

The entire first year of a fellowship is meant to be difficult, a time for learning protocols, treatments, and procedures, and gaining experience in the tactical world of executing clinical and research plans. The inpatient service months were arduous, split between a busy bone marrow–transplant unit and a shared inpatient/consult service for oncology patients. The learning curve was steep, with every day bringing new challenges, new questions, and hours upon hours of seeking new answers. Catching up never seemed possible, as there was always some person or some patient there to remind me of everything I still didn't know, while I continually felt like I was teetering on the precipice of abject failure. Feeling inadequate, I longed for any form of validation from a decade of working in medicine, but the validation never seemed to come.

The long weeks of seeing patients in the hospital were accompanied by phone calls at home at every hour of the night. At a large academic institution, this sometimes means receiving calls every twenty to thirty minutes, all night long. I remember getting a phone call at 2 a.m. from France for a routine update on a patient referral. Fortunately, the communication was in English, as four years of high school French were not at the front of my mind while I was half-awake in the middle of the night.

I thought, *Merci beaucoup, my Parisian colleague, but next time remember our clinic opens at 8 a.m.*

For physicians, no regulations exist to limit home-based work hours, so the following day I trudged into work after only an hour of sleep. From my first steps in the door, there were normal expectations for a normal day, and no room for excuses. After working another long shift, I rubbed my weary eyes as my head slowly started to nod. The clock on the workroom wall read 7 p.m., and I thought about the cumulative circuits of the clock since I last fell into a slumber.

With a debilitated mind, I drove home from work—but I didn't make it very far. A few miles from the house, I rounded a curve and my eyes closed for a moment too long. By the time my eyes startled open again, the damage was already done. In a jarring detour off the asphalt, my car crashed into a (thankfully unoccupied) vehicle parked on the side of the road.

A few days later, the insurance agent claimed the car was totaled. I survived physically unscathed, with a convenient $6,000 get-out-of-work-for-a-day absence note. Having escaped serious injury, I reminded myself that if I could just get through the year, all the hard work would be done, and next year I would be able to practice medicine the way I had always hoped.

The months working in the inpatient hospital units kept coming, and the daily processes buried me deeper in a hole, away from any connection to a purpose. Every once in a while I would connect to a patient and their family, and then the month would be over and I would abandon them and head back to another busy service, clinic, or basic science laboratory. I had long since recognized that in academic medicine, every student, resident, and fellow moved to a different part of the hospital every month, with a new set of duties and responsibilities. For each new rotation I had another hat to wear, another steep learning curve to climb, and another set of unrelenting expectations to meet. I started to feel like I didn't know who I was, because I had to be someone different every time the calendar page turned.

The moments with patients offered a glimpse of what I was hoping for in medicine: to connect to people, share in their stories, and help them navigate their illness. But every time, there were abrupt stops and awkward ends to any evolving rapport. It often felt like a direct fracturing of the relationship, handing patients off to another person in what became a routine, "things left unsaid" breakup, and I dreaded this process every single time. I would try to spend time reconnecting while on other rotations, or at the end of a day, but the moment, the rapport, and the relationship always felt tarnished in some way. I felt as though I was not there for them when they needed me most, and the shame of missing Zoe's death crept back into my life again.

There were good times as well, mostly with a newfound friend and mentor, Dr. Ray Barfield. Ray was a former stem cell–transplant physician from St. Jude Medical Center and a philosopher, writer, musician, and theologian. At the time that we met, he was teaching himself to play guitar and writing a book of poetry. Ray held appointments at both the medical and divinity schools, which is rare in modern medicine. A true outside-the-box thinker, he was focused on holistic healing while helping other people cope with their suffering. When I picture the famous nineteenth-century painting *The Doctor* by Luke Fildes, I imagine Ray, without the whiskers and stiff collar of the physician depicted in the image, sitting patiently at a child's bedside, deep in contemplation.

On one of our first inpatient services working together, Ray and I took care of a young man in the ICU who was critically ill from lymphoma. Andre was a big kid, over six feet tall and 270 pounds, and he was angry and embarrassed about his hospitalization. According to the nurses, he had first felt ill while swimming off the Outer Banks of North Carolina a few days prior to his admission to the hospital. For weeks, he believed the ocean caused his illness. I would have loved to discuss this theory with him, and tried to educate him about his condition and how we were planning to treat it, but he refused to speak with anyone. Andre defiantly avoided even simple questions and answers.

On subsequent visits, both Ray and I tried to engage him in conversation. He just stared at the wall with a look of disgust on his face as the stonewalling continued. The following day, on morning rounds, I concocted a plan that I proposed to Ray—a bit of medical theater to provoke a reaction.

Andre was lying in bed in his corner room of the oncology unit, a room staff knew to only visit with good reason. Andre had seemed to want it that way, and I am sure he would have hung a "Do Not Enter" sign on the door frame had the hospital allowed it. The lights were off and the blinds shut while he lay there, staring at his phone. In the near-total darkness, all I saw was a face softly lit by a cell phone's glow. Ray and I walked into the room together, sat next to Andre's bed, turned on the TV, and just sat there in silence—a beautiful, prolonged, awkward silence. We sat and waited.

After about forty-five minutes, Andre finally looked up from his phone and asked, "What are you guys doing here?"

We replied, "Just watching TV. Is that okay?"

He begrudgingly answered, "Well, you didn't even ask first . . . but I guess."

He cracked a smile then, and we knew we had broken through his tough exterior. We waited him out, letting him know we weren't going anywhere and would walk this journey with him. In the days to come, it became clear that Andre's pushing people away was a defense mechanism to manage brewing anxiety and depression.

As I stepped out of his room, I noticed a cart full of isolation masks—those lower-face coverings medical personnel wear to prevent the spread of respiratory infection—sitting outside his door. I knew he didn't put them there, but the irony of the name "isolation" echoed through my mind. A few steps further, I stripped off the visage of the healthy, happy, and well-adjusted physician. As I walked off the oncology floor, a confident stride turned into a despondent shuffle, and then I sat alone, in the false comfort of my own profound isolation.

I was already sleep deprived and feeling overworked, and the cumulative impact of caring for other people continued to grow every day. For a decade, the heaviness of story after story of human suffering stuck with me. I never forgot those patients and families under my care, and my internal scale was tipping. Each step forward became more painful to take.

When a week of vacation came, I hoped for a momentary reprieve from the never-ending grind. In a depressed mind-set, I headed with Lauren to Disney World, the "Happiest Place on Earth." We watched fireworks, ate dinner at the Cinderella Castle, and rode the teacups in an innocent search for any reconciliation with joy. On the Jungle Cruise ride, I remember cracking a smile at "the back side of water" jokes, while briefly feeling a boat-sized weight being lifted off me. In the park, we walked through fairy tale after fairy tale, and yet I still sensed an unhappily-ever-after looming.

Two days into the trip, we stood in line for the Animal Kingdom's Dinosaur ride. When we were close to the front, my phone rang with a call from a colleague. I immediately recalled the collegial wrath I had sustained a few weeks before, when I failed to answer an overnight email before the morning alarm clock sounded. Resigned to meeting the expectations of the medical culture, I had to answer. Steps from the turnstile entrance, I accepted the call.

"Adam, the bone marrow biopsy results are back on your patient," a rushed voice stated.

"Okay . . ." I trailed off, confused, in my vacation frame of mind. A long silence followed.

"The family is waiting for the results, so why don't you call them and let them know."

In an indoctrinated obedience, I stepped out of the line.

Now, sitting on a bench outside the ride, under the jaws of a ferocious beast, I was back on my phone. Moments from enjoying an exhilarating "thrill ride," I had been detoured onto a different roller coaster altogether. As a jovial group of teens walked out of the gift shop and children laughed in the background, I dialed a number to devastate a young family.

Out of the corner of my eye, I observed water trickling down the edge of a nearby fountain, and then heard the tearful drops on the other end of the line. While speaking to a mother, I felt the tears stolen from her sense of maternal joy, sinking us both deeper into an uncertainty about our futures. As we talked, I started to walk, and before long I found myself standing at the base of the Tree of Life sculpture, with Lauren a few steps away. I had hoped for relief, a release—just a momentary reprieve from the gravity of my work. Instead, I hung up the phone and a tear streamed down my left cheek. I looked up at the towering timber monument, as leaf-filled branches celebrated spring's renewal of life. But as the phone held onto an echo of the word "cancer," I found myself standing in the encroaching darkness of a perennial shadow.

After that first year, as a second-year fellow, I expected to receive fewer calls, enjoy more sleep, and have a stronger voice in the process. The long-promised rewards of practicing medicine the way I had always hoped to were finally on the way. I thought, *In what other career do you have to wait twelve years before making any decisions on your own?* Still, I waited patiently for that moment, and the moment never came. My opinions still didn't seem to matter. I was still at the bottom of the totem pole. The lack of change led to a spiraling recurrence of depression. I fell into the void of a relentless nothing brought about by nothing changing. The sleep was still sporadic, and the cumulative weight of unsolvable problems became too much to bear. It was during this time that I began to lose my identity. I could not answer the question, *Why did I go into medicine?*

I was trained to tie my worth to academic success and medical achievement, and because of that, I no longer recognized the man in the mirror enough to know if I was asking the right person. In the disillusion, all I saw was a shell of a person staring back at me. I was apathetic about daily tasks and started caring less about the important things in my life, and less still about anything else. Trapped in meaningless cycles, I felt disconnected from any greater purpose I had previously enjoyed.

Luckily for me, I found a solution right around the corner.

I thought back to the time when, sitting in a college classroom, I heard the harrowing words of a middle-aged pharmacist: relief, release, warmth, and numb. I worked a normal day, put on a brave face, and then went home. But his words continued to resonate: relief, release, warmth, numb. The words took me back to the sensation I had felt in college of an anxiety defused by alcohol, the feelings of chaos from an emotional discord being quieted.

At work, I often sat across a table from anxious patients and parents and shared the news of a poor chance of survival. At home, I sat at the kitchen table, telling myself the same thing. In my resignation, I started to have a couple of drinks to numb the growing unease in my life. I took the first drink to ease the pain of witnessing years of patients' suffering, and the second to lighten the load of the decades of my own. And it worked, temporarily quieting the tornadic cycles of unstable emotions churned up by a life filled with guilt, insecurity, inadequacy, and trauma.

In the midst of an untreated depression, I had a single drink at night, and then two. If you have walked into an Alcoholics Anonymous meeting, sat in the corner, and listened, the rest of the story will sound familiar. Within a few weeks, I didn't feel as though two drinks provided the calming effect I desired, so two soon became three, and then four. I also drank earlier and earlier after leaving work, consumed more in less time, and eventually started to fall asleep before the sun set. I didn't have a reason to stay awake, because the state of sleep was also an escape.

In a conscious calculation, I made sure never to neglect or jeopardize my work or my patients, and when I was on call, I would simply go without alcohol. The nights on call were when I should have realized

I was relying on alcohol as my only coping mechanism, because I was miserable. I actually had to face the problems in my life, the strains and stressors, the internal monologue, and I did not have the ability to handle it. I continued to work and function, but I started distancing myself from Lauren, friends, and family. My best friend and I did not talk for months as I continued to drink more and do less, and within a short amount of time I began to feel the physical effects of the abuse.

One Saturday afternoon, a few months into the downward spiral, Lauren found me passed out, facedown in the woods behind our house. I remember tasting a gritty saltiness as a dog's tongue startled me awake and Lauren stood over me in utter disbelief. Our Labrador retriever's panting grin seemed to infuriate her, as her feelings deviated greatly from the dog's. In the same space, I felt the presence of unconditional love from one and piercing judgment from the other. Without a word, or any concept of time of space, I walked back inside with the dog, on a paw-traced path of least resistance. I stumbled into bed, and then woke up early the following morning with an overwhelming urge to have another drink. Lauren met me in the kitchen, asking where I had left the car keys, but I didn't even know where to begin. It felt like a trap, and I was immediately defensive. I didn't reply, and she didn't want me to.

She snapped, "I looked for them for five hours in the woods last night with a flashlight, and finally found them. Here you go, you're welcome."

I felt small, embarrassed, and helpless—more reasons to have another drink.

I ran away from the unease of the personal conflict, owing to a conflict-avoidance habit ingrained in me from an early age. More specifically, I drove toward a familiar location: the liquor store parking lot.

Do you know what it's like to sit in a liquor store parking lot early in the morning, waiting for the clerk to unlock the front doors? It's an irrepressible collision of guilt with an unwillingness to accept the severity of a problem.

A few times I managed to drive away for a couple of hours, only to return with less guilt and a feeling of accomplishment for having survived for a bit more time without another drink. Yet instead of coming to terms with the problems mounting in my life, I did have another drink, and then another. A few days later, I found myself falling down an entire flight of stairs at our house, and then laughing about it. I learned to do that at an early age, as hallway trips and arm punches always seemed funny to other people. I laughed to mask the pain growing deep inside, a pain outwardly revealed in a serious bruise that covered the length of my entire hip for almost three weeks. Alcoholics tend to bruise easily, and this was the first sign of an imbalance in my liver and blood, a marker of the progressive illness consuming me.

I convinced myself that it was normal; I fell, I bruised, it healed. Now on to the next drink. After several more weeks of living in this pattern, I slightly injured my knee playing a pickup game of basketball. Needless to say, the shots of vodka before I took the court may have been a contributing factor. Yet I suffered only a minor scrape, not worthy of anything more than a superficial dressing. I went home and went to bed, and the following afternoon, a Saturday, I found myself sitting on the couch with a throbbing pain around my knee. I unwrapped the dressing, looked down, and felt an unusual warmth over the tender, swollen joint. I attempted to drain the fluid, took some antibiotics left over from a dental procedure, and carried on with my weekend.

Physicians are really good at self-medication.

The following morning, I woke up to see that the wound was clearly getting worse. For a few hours I tried to contact Lauren, but my calls went unanswered. As I dialed one more time, the redness of the wound streaked up my leg, inch by inch, all the way to my thigh. In the medical world, this is known as streaking lymphangitis. Fancy names aside, the term means the infection was traveling quickly throughout my body. If my Parisian colleague were still on the phone, he would have said, "*Pas bien*"—no good, a rapid sign of a serious, spreading, and potentially life-threatening infection.

By this time I was lightheaded, feverish, and feeling uneasy, so I knew I needed medical attention fast. One final time, I reached Lauren's voicemail. Reluctantly, then, I called one of my bosses. He lived a few blocks away and I knew he would answer the phone.

"Andrew, I'm not feeling well at all. I need to head to the hospital," I frantically said.

"Okay. What do you need from me?"

"Please come over. I can't drive."

He could sense the panic in my voice, so he rushed over immediately, and we headed to the hospital. When we arrived, the nurses saw the paleness in my face and rushed me through intake.

Having my boss push me in a wheelchair into the hospital where I work is an experience I never want to go through again. I knew the whole reason I was in this predicament was that alcoholism depletes the immune system. It was yet another physical manifestation of the extent of my disease. My body was weak, getting frailer by the drink, without an ability to fight off the rapidly spreading infection.

Soon afterward, Lauren showed up at the hospital and we mostly sat in silence. I sat in a quiet but knowing frame of mind, jarred from months of denial, but I kept it all to myself because of the shame that was growing exponentially with every attempted IV stick.

I stayed in the hospital for two days, receiving antibiotics and a surgical drainage while having orthopedic, infectious disease, and surgery consults from people I knew peripherally. In an observation room in the back of the hospital, a simple drape and flimsy gown provided little cover for my surreptitious life. With every pullback of the curtain, I saw a rising apprehension in the faces that recognized the fragility of my state. I feared my medical chart would confirm suspicions of my secret use, as the foundation of an early career cracked and crumbled underneath my feet. Hour by hour, I waited for the initial cracks to appear, but there was a welcome silence in the hospital halls. I slept through it, and when I woke, I felt reassured that I could remain hidden in the shadows.

The following day, imaging studies were used to ensure the infection was not spreading into the knee joint, and the final infectious disease workup yielded a methicillin-resistant staphylcoccus aureus (MRSA) infection. MRSA is a serious bacterium that, if not treated appropriately, can be life-threatening; a MRSA infection can be fatal even when appropriately treated—a sobering thought, I imagine, even for people in a healthy state of mind.

I was lucky, as I physically recovered and was discharged from the hospital. The incision healed over a short period of time, but my pride did not. I revisited the emotional pain I felt as a young man lying in the street with a tennis regionals match only a few days away, and the wounds of shame only grew deeper. I should have learned a lesson, but my ongoing emotional distress far outweighed the physical scare, so I went back to the bottle, and a few short weeks later, I would find myself sitting under an ash tree in a state park, forty-five minutes from home, with a pair of bottles and a plan to never come home.

In the days after the hospital discharge, I barely ate, yet I went to work with a faux smile, braved the day, and then drove straight to the liquor store after work. I knew all the stores on the way home, as by this time I was drinking every night. Over time, the serving size of Smirnoff's went from a half pint to a pint, and eventually to a fifth. I consciously rotated the stores so that none of the cashiers would recognize me as the guy buying alcohol every day. Secrecy was an exhausting mental exercise. I remember feeling a sense of panic one night when I recognized the clerk in one of the stores from the day before, when she was at a different location. She also worked at one of the stores closer to home, but presumably had been called to fill in at the other store that night.

She nodded at me, and her expression said, "I know you, but I'm not sure from where."

I avoided eye contact, paid for the bottle, and left, but I still felt mortified and obsessed about the coincidence for days. Moments like that forced me to face the reality of my addiction, even if for a brief moment, and I couldn't live with those emotions—they felt too real, too heavy, and too demeaning. Which made me want another drink.

I drove home and sat in the car in the garage, contemplating whether or not I should even go inside. By this point Lauren knew I was struggling, and it was easier just to hide, because her love felt confrontational, and I just wanted to be left alone. She would try to reach out, and I would just sit in the garage or on the patio behind our home. I would drink alone in those spaces, being quietly and mindfully unassuming. To her it was always clear what was happening, but even though she did her best to fight for me, I felt like I was already gone.

I hid liquor bottles all over the house—in garage cabinets, in book bags, and under a mattress in the spare bedroom. I was a secretive, closet drinker. I never went out to restaurants or bars, as I preferred to be alone. I thought I was cleverly camouflaging the deepest parts of my suffering, as I had learned to do in college when no one really knew when I was drinking.

Yet my spouse's uncovering of this secret life abruptly crippled my perceptions, and I was not ready to hear the truth. I continued to find new hiding spaces and to push those closest to me further away. Lauren watched the slow-moving train wreck for months, in all of its painful and unsettling destruction. One evening she got home from work to find me lying in bed, under the covers, at 5:30 p.m. She worked up the courage to lie down next to me. I had intentionally chosen vodka for moments like this, to minimize the risk of her smelling it on me. Yet the odor permeated the down comforter, and she could sense the dragon waiting in his cave with 100-proof breath.

I spent weekends, and some weeknights, out on a golf course, and I don't really even like golf. It was the perfect escape from personal judgments, and it gave me time alone with my closest friend—the bottle. I golfed for the time I could spend in silence, for the zero expectations, and as an escape from the ramifications of what my life had become. I did not keep score; that was never the point. On one such outing, I had slipped out of work at the end of the day to hit the course on a late Wednesday afternoon, and at the first tee a disheveled man approached me. He wore sweatpants and a stained T-shirt, with his belly protruding where the T-shirt ended.

"Looking for someone to play with?" he asked in a Southern drawl.

Avoiding an awkward moment, I answered, "I guess, why not?" It just felt easier to say yes.

We joined each other on the course. He was in his late fifties and "retired." It became readily apparent that his mission was similar to mine. By the time we reached the first fairway his bottle of whiskey was already open. I concealed my vodka in a Gatorade bottle until about the fourth hole, when we began openly drinking together. We didn't speak much. In a silent understanding of our alcoholism, we knew the point was to drink together, not alone, while never acknowledging aloud the depths of our mutual truth. Later on in the round, I grew uneasy in the realization that I was staring at my own possible fate. It was a "Ghost of Christmas Future" moment, a dark reveal of how my struggles might continue to play out. I saw myself divorced, middle-aged, unemployed, and lonely, while still consumed by the temptation of another bottle. But I also knew I probably wouldn't survive long enough to see such wreckage. These thoughts were almost immediately sobering, and I left the course abruptly in the middle of the eleventh fairway. Without any explanation, without any social accommodation or polite cue, I simply vanished from his sight, and from the recognition of what my life had become.

The following week, I nestled my car within the yellow lines of a gun store parking lot. Seeing the potential for years of alcoholic turmoil ahead, I decided I wouldn't let my life go on that long.

CHAPTER SEVEN

Into the Woods

Walking out of the gun store, I sensed an ironic form of rejection, thinking that I couldn't even kill myself without causing a hassle. Back to the car and then the garage, I had a few more shots of vodka, and the visions of closing the garage with the car engine running came calling once more.

As the sun rose the following morning, I woke up and decided I could no longer wait for a gun license or endure a holding period. The dreams of making a positive impact in other people's lives were gone. I had failed at being a son, failed at being a husband, and failed as a physician. All I could think about was relieving other people from the burden of my presence in their lives.

I resigned myself to the woods.

The woods had always been a place of peace, a place to not be seen, a place to get lost in without trails or paths to judge how I had gone off track. The woods were also a place I would not easily be found in. I often fantasized about escaping into the woods, living out *My Side of the Mountain*, my favorite childhood book. The story's young hero carved out a new life for himself in the woods after abandoning his old ways. He made new woodland friends, built himself a home, and learned a new way of taking care of himself in an uncertain world. In essence, the book was about survival. I just wished it could be that simple and innocent for me.

I trudged into the woods, over crackling twigs and slippery thistle, and found a moment of peace under a tree, sitting and sipping and thinking. I planned to drink myself to death with the help of a bottle of sleeping pills.

After months of suicidal thoughts, vaguely developed plans, and prior attempts to explore the end of my own life, I realized the simplest answer was in the medicine cabinet all along. In truth, the means didn't really matter to me anyway, only the end.

I pondered where it had all gone so violently wrong as I sat there beneath the tree, in deep contemplation about how happy everyone would be without the nuisance of me in their lives and the gratitude the world would feel when I was gone. I could not muster the energy to carve my name into a tree trunk, or make even a single mark. In my mind this was fitting. My mark had never been made.

No goodbye letter, either; I had nothing meaningful to say.

There I sat underneath a billowing ash tree, in a secluded portion of Eno River State Park, with the babbling sounds of water rushing over rocks nearby. If I took you there, you would admire the majesty of the spot in all its pristine beauty. What I heard, though, was the mocking chirps of a family of sparrows, taunting me to go ahead and end it. I listened to the wind rustling leaves, a sound that transformed into a chorus of whispered negativities from my past. And I concentrated on the incessant flow of water as a reminder of the life draining out of me.

I looked across a field at a misplaced boulder nestled into the bank of the river. It was a jagged, misshapen rock that didn't seem to belong there because it created a turbulence of white water around it. I saw the river and rock at war with each other, the rock acting as an unnecessary and intrusive barrier to a smooth flow downstream.

So, I walked over to the river's edge and climbed on top of the rocky shelf. For a moment it felt good not to be alone, as I felt connected with the rock, each of us eroding under a continual pressure. It felt like we were both inconvenient weights, disrupting and disturbing life all around us, slowly drowning in our misguided ways.

The view down the river was a peaceful one in contrast to the chaos of my mental state. It was a quiet, hidden space where I hoped to find a final resting place. I didn't think far beyond that moment, as I honestly didn't see the point. I would be gone, and the world would be better off without me.

What did the rest matter, anyway?

Hours went by as I replayed memories of some of the greatest disappointments of my life in consecutive order. I didn't speak, but often caught myself shaking my head, with maybe a few mumbles under my breath.

Between grumblings, I flashed back to my cowardly failures to complete the looming deed. Months before, I had sat on a bathroom floor behind a locked door, with a paring knife in hand. Minute after minute, I pricked my skin in a sensationalized test of whatever feelings may have remained in me. I turned on the water and visualized the dilution of the blood from an opened vessel into scattered hues of red, and then pink, as my life circled down the drain. I saw in the splashed droplets a beautiful release of what was once inner suffering out into the world. In a heartbeat rhythm, each drop ticked down the remaining moments of a wasted life. As I envisioned the aftermath, I ran the knife, blade side down, along the hairs of my forearm. In reality, the sharp edge never left an outward scar, as the severest cuts remained deep within. Regardless of the depth of the cuts, I never forgot how I felt in those moments: for the first time in a long time, I felt as though I was finally the one in control.

After a few more flashbacks, I pictured a stadium full of people in a standing ovation, cheering my absence. I saw ticker tape parades and fireworks, a sort of self-deprecating narcissism, I suppose, as I imagined that people cared enough to celebrate my departure. I cracked a smile at the thought of it, anyway—probably the first time I had genuinely smiled in months.

I knew that I wouldn't feel bullied anymore, and people wouldn't have to look after me any longer, either. Best of all, I would no longer have to live a life removed from the person I had always wanted to be.

After a few more ironic smiles, I sank deeper into pangs of guilt. As I reflected on the plight of those patients who had fought hard to overcome their diseases, I could not reconcile the disconnect between their tenacity and my state of resignation. I pondered the personal characteristics that gave them the ability to come out stronger on the other side. The guilt consumed me, not for those I would leave behind, but for the patients who lost their lives to their diseases after heroic battles, while I didn't even have an inclination to fight.

For most of the afternoon I sat under the tree, soaking up self-hatred. I contemplated when the appropriate time would be to take the thirty pills and be done with it. As evening approached, I poured them into an eager palm. Over and over, I transferred a pill at a time from one hand to the other, calculating and counting a dose, and I weighed the gravity of an irreversible decision. I sat in wonder, noting how millions of times a simple swallow was instinctual, benign, and forgotten. Grounded in a new reality, I felt the saliva in my mouth, and the power of nature's mechanism of mortality. Conscious of every breath I took, and then every swallow, I counted the seconds remaining in my life. As I took another swig of vodka, I closed a fist around dozens of pills, leaned my head back against the cold, damp bark of a tree, and sighed.

Moments from action, I wrestled with the thought of a final hand-to-mouth maneuver, but instead sensed a rustling under my legs. Though I had been numb to the world for months, I felt something again, an unnatural stirring. Then I heard it, underneath a small patch of leaves. I looked down at my phone as it vibrated for a few seconds longer, and then the screen went dark. I stared down at it, jarred from my state of resignation, and then, seconds later, it started to vibrate again. After months of disconnections and dial tones, Lauren called a second time, and then a third.

On the fourth call, I answered. By grace, her love had waited me out. "Mind joining me for dinner tonight?" she asked in a casual tone.

I just listened.

"I would love it if you would just come home."

The Hollywood ending would be that Lauren came to pick me up in those woods and we lived happily ever after. In that version, I would go from being moments away from taking my own life to being hoisted onto shoulders, taking a long walk out of the woods back into the world a happy man. But Hollywood is convenient that way. The truth is that I crawled out of the woods on my hands and knees, through mud puddles of personal misery. As I was well off the trail, it took two hours for her to even find me, and when she did, I sensed that she wished she hadn't. With a pocketful of pills and an empty vodka bottle, I collapsed into the backseat of her car, on the verge of an alcoholic blackout.

This is where the long journey into recovery began—the journey to reclaim my soul, my identity, my purpose, and my meaning, and to find a way to grow into the person I always wanted to be. Forget medicine; this was about reclaiming my life by finding a way to live well in a world turned upside down.

The next few days were painstaking, and shame prevented me from looking Lauren in the eyes. Newly vulnerable, I sat terrified and alone in the darkest of holes, with the vicious demons of addiction hovering around me. Just as she had in our childhood, my sister chased after me, stride after supportive stride. And to protect their son, my parents laid out their love, yielding a hope that I was worthy of being saved. With Lauren, my parents, and Amanda supporting me, I met with a very compassionate psychiatrist and counselor. I restarted the medication for depression, joined an Alcoholics Anonymous program, and began the meticulous work of self-discovery, opening up new wounds before old ones could heal.

I voluntarily disclosed the treatment to my employer and was mandated to enroll in a professional-assistance program for physicians. And day by day, I continued to feel miserable. I merely existed hour by hour, and sometimes moment by moment. For days, the physical abstinence felt like the worst flu symptoms I could have imagined. For weeks, and then months, the emotional cravings continuously called, reminding me that I could end the symptoms at any instant with a short drive and a clear plastic bottle.

As part of the recovery process, I met with a community-based primary care doctor, truly hoping the worst parts were in the past. Although it felt impossible at times, I had a plan to move forward. The primary care doctor was an older gentleman with a comb-over hairstyle and a peppering of black hair amid all of the gray. He spoke in a measured countenance, with a welcome Southern charm. I noticed a wall plastered with Ivy League diplomas, the accreditations of a career defined by medals, ribbons, and professional validations bestowed by other people. He struck me as one of those physicians who never retires, just continues to work until the final days of his life, having never developed any other hobbies, passions, or interests beyond the clinic walls. From friends outside of medicine, I had heard about the way he approached their medical conditions with kindness, and I hoped to receive a similar level of gentle acceptance.

But a perplexing thing happened, leading me to question every decision I had made in the previous few days, and it left me feeling isolated, angry, and regretful for seeking help. To this day, it has served as an impetus for me to speak out publicly about my recovery. The doctor bluntly asked me, "Do you really want to do this?"

I had disclosed to this individual my feelings of depression, suicidal thoughts, and alcohol use to cope with a brutal unease about my life. And now this question?

"Do you really want to do this?"

At first, I did not understand the question. Should I have explored other options? Was I going about this the wrong way? I thought I was doing the right thing and was on a path to reclaim my life, but had I made a terrible mistake?

It became clear that he was not asking whether I still wanted to go into treatment. He was not questioning whether I really wanted to feel better and start fresh and have a chance at a healthy, productive life in recovery. The doctor meant, "Are you sure you want help for *these* conditions, which may mean publicly disclosing your treatment to a medical society that will shame you for it?"

I could not believe this physician was actually asking if I wanted to just turn around, walk out, and not speak of my issues again—words spoken to a person just a few weeks removed from a trip to the woods with a plan to die. Why would someone ever second-guess an individual in the midst of a life-or-death crisis?

I felt a shock of anxiety tingle down my spine and the gravity of shame forced my eyes down to the ground. The implications were that I would never be treated the same way again. As soon the physician made this statement, I realized it had already begun.

Years later, I would understand the complexities of his warning, but in my moment of suffering, it disturbed me to my core. Unfortunately, I found that these considerations come into play more frequently than I could have imagined, inside and outside the halls of medicine.

Several years into recovery, I spoke at a community event for professionals in higher education. Before the talk, a young instructor walked up to me and said, "I wanted to take time away for mental health treatment, but the bar for reentry is incredibly high."

Hearing this drew me back to those initial moments of my own recovery.

"I was encouraged to hide my history of bipolar disease," she added. "They thought that would be better, for the safety of the students."

This is what we do with mental health conditions: we immediately link them to the potential harm they can do to other people.

A few months later, after a lecture I gave on the East Coast, a resident physician asked if we could talk for a few minutes. We found a quiet room, and he started inquiring about my experience, but the look in his eyes suggested that he was holding something back, something he wanted to share but was afraid to reveal. I will never forget the pained expression on his face; it's the look we in the medical culture have created by terrifying individuals into not seeking professional help. His eyes conveyed a fear of retribution, shame, distrust, and career ruin. I told him we were in a safe space; anything he said would remain confidential. We could just talk.

He began to cry.

He said, "A lot of your story is my story. I work functionally, but I struggle on and off with depression, so I have three or four drinks a night to fall asleep."

He said he had made benign inquiries to a few colleagues about the resources available for counseling, and the message he received was always the same: do not disclose anything unless absolutely necessary because it will destroy your career.

I counseled him some more, offered my contact information as a building block for his support network, encouraged him to seek therapy, and offered to speak with his administrators while standing by his side. We still stay in touch, and this young soul has trudged along his own road toward a happier destiny. But honestly, if we cannot change the look in that young man's eyes, or rather the fear that brought it on in the first place, we will never make the medical culture accepting of individuals with mental health and addiction stories.

Despite the warnings, I said yes to treatment.

For the rest of my career, I knew I would see paperwork littered with questions such as, "Have you ever been treated for a mental health condition?" I resolved to start checking the "yes" boxes on all such employment applications and medical licensing and hospital credentialing forms.

Yes, I have a history of alcoholism.

Yes, I have been in mental health treatment.

Yes, I have been on medications for depression.

Ironically, yes, I am alive to check these boxes at all.

As of writing this book, a vast majority of hospitals, state medical licensing bodies, and insurance credentialing agencies still require these questions (and more) to be answered when applying for a job. The presence of the questions alone deters people from seeking help that could save their lives. I answered them, and I lived, but the ongoing suicide epidemic in medicine suggests that these questions contribute to the deaths of medical professionals every single day.

I like to think that I did not say yes, exactly, but that yes happened to me. Because the truth is, had I known exactly how I would be treated in the first several years of recovery, I would never have entered treatment voluntarily. I would have declined the help and I would probably have died, becoming just another statistic in the growing epidemic of suicide. In recovery, I think about all the people at this same crossroads who are forced into no-win decisions of either treatment and punishment, or another way out altogether.

I often think of those individuals who sit in the same chair I had, and about the gravity of their single yes or no. I think of those who didn't survive, and how we need to approach this disclosure–and–treatment process differently. The status quo clearly isn't working, and in the face of an ongoing national crisis, a lot more honey and less vinegar is needed to attract people into life-saving treatment.

After I said yes to treatment, I did not immediately start to feel better. In fact, the first six months of treatment proved to be incredibly difficult. I was sober, on an antidepressant, going to meetings and counseling, in a physician-assisted drug-monitoring program, and building my support network—yet things were not getting better. During that time I felt like the world had taken away the one coping skill I had, so I was just as miserable as I had been before. Maybe even more so at times. Alcohol was the one tool I knew that worked without fail. The emotional wounds were always there, but I had been numb to them. Now they were really starting to hurt. I realized it was time for a radical dissection of the old me to uncover my true identity.

With this realization and about six months of sobriety, I started to find a fresh perspective and a newfound peace—but an impending emotional wreck was waiting right around the corner.

CHAPTER EIGHT

Exile

A year into recovery I completed my final projects, and my oncology fellowship officially ended. I wrapped up the clinical workload and said my goodbyes to patients and colleagues. One family gave me a framed picture of their son, a survivor of leukemia, as a lasting testament to his courageous victory over his disease. The picture sits on my bookshelf today as a daily reminder of the meaningful work I still have left to do. Lauren and I packed up the picture frame and our other belongings in cardboard boxes, and just like that, the next chapter of our lives was about to begin.

Our intention was to move back to Indianapolis, where Lauren had secured a job as a clinical research coordinator for an orthopedic trauma team. Lauren is one of those hardworking, behind-the-scenes people in medicine who work diligently so that medical teams can enroll patients in clinical trials for new and innovative modes of treatment. With her continued love and support, I planned to spend the following year working as a hospitalist (a physician who assumes the care of hospitalized patients in the place of their primary care physicians) until a slot opened for a palliative medicine fellowship the following July.

Late in the fall, we settled into our new Indianapolis neighborhood, relishing the reunification with family and old friends. We bought a modest house on a quiet cul-de-sac with a wide-open green space behind it. Our home, laid out north to south, had a picturesque view that paralleled the dawning of the next chapter of our lives. I started working at the hospital in early November, but was still waiting for final credentialing paperwork before I could officially see patients. For over a month I worked on smaller projects, going through administrative processes while waiting for hospital credential approval.

As the snow fell on a mid-December day, we hung Christmas stockings over the fireplace and prepared for a season of family celebrations. Life was starting to take shape. It felt like a fresh new beginning for our lives together. We talked for the first time about having kids, raising a family, and other long-term goals. We connected with local support groups and felt as though we finally belonged somewhere after the tumultuous events of the prior years. Day by day, I gained confidence in my recovery and felt as though I finally had my feet on sturdy ground.

Then, twelve days before Christmas, I received a phone call to my direct office line. It was the administrative assistant to the chairman of pediatrics.

"Can you come up to the chairman's office right away, please?"

A sinking feeling settled into the pit of my stomach. This was an unexpected sense of foreboding, but I knew exactly what was about to happen.

Head down, I trudged up the back stairwell, five long sets of stairs. Back in elementary school, I used to count each step in my head to distract from the anxiety of having once been shoved down a similar flight. So, I counted to ten, then started over, and finally, with an eight, nine, ten, I arrived outside the chairman's office and was ushered right in.

It was a short meeting with a shockingly brief reveal.

The chairman's suite was a corner office with a bank of windows on one wall and a leather couch in the corner. As I took a few steps toward the corner, memories flooded back of sitting in a waiting room outside a pair of locked steel hospital doors, waiting for approval to access the healing process inside.

The chairman said, "We won't be able to hire you because your credentialing was not approved."

He went on, but my attention shifted to a lump growing in my throat. I felt a tightening grasp of hands stronger than mine impeding the passage of every single breath.

I melted into the depths of the leather coach and did not utter a single word. I briefly glanced out the window at the view of the sprawling medical campus I was deemed unworthy of joining. The subtext was that the credentialing process focused on my history of addiction, and not the recovery. Without broader inquiry, the process was stymied by stamps of disapproval, one mental health checked box at a time. On the forms, no space was provided for words like "successful," "voluntary," or "better physician because of it." I paused as a tear welled deep within and my head sank even lower, the pride of a successful early recovery having immediately vanished.

"Thank you for the opportunity," was all I could think to say.

My heart was broken, and I felt immediately transported back to those thoughts I had in the woods.

You are not good enough.

You should have done more.

Not long afterward, a familiar pattern unfolded. Guilt, shame, resentment, and anger.

I was living the family physician's prophecy that I would lose future career opportunities by disclosing my mental health struggles.

I called Lauren, and then plodded back down the stairwell to tell my division chief the news. It was surreal, but she was kind as I handed over my badge and office keys. Just like that, without fanfare, without incident, and with over a year of successful recovery under my belt, it was done.

I sat in my car in the parking garage for over an hour as the engine ran and the exhaust fumes revived a not-so-distant recollection. Then I drove home, in the middle of the day, past six different liquor stores. I took notice of every neon sign. I felt the steering wheel nudge, as though it was driving me back to a reliable comfort. In the rising tide of uncontrollable anguish, the simplest solution is always regression—two steps backward into a self-medicated haven, to guard against the onslaught of negative emotions. Relapse would have been so easy.

The next few days were a blur, as I was officially unemployed and, in my catastrophic internal monologue, seemingly unemployable. Not six weeks prior, we had purchased a new home and moved across the country for this opportunity. I spent the next several days on the phone, reaching out to old connections and working with a professional physician recruiter, as there were bills to pay and a family to support. I felt trapped in a devolving career, with two thousand dollars a month of loan repayments and 250k in medical school debt hanging over my head.

I was forced to navigate the minefields of the business of medicine as well. Most hospitals make their doctors sign noncompete clauses, so if I took a temporary job locally, I would be barred from accepting any other opportunity to work in pediatrics. Most noncompete clauses don't allow transfer of employment to another institution within a certain geographic radius (usually 50 to 100 miles) for a set amount of time (one to two years). So, taking a temporary job in Indianapolis could limit my options for several years. I had to broaden the search to protect any future chance to crawl back into academic medicine, while still being hamstrung by the fact that every state requires individual medical licensing, which can sometimes take six to eight months, or even longer for someone with a history like mine.

My father offered to connect me with the pediatric physicians' group in my hometown. I knew most of those people already—the CMO of the hospital was the father of an old high school friend—but this sounded humiliating, as the last thing I wanted to do was bring my baggage back to my hometown and air dirty laundry in front of people I had known my entire life. I feared those people would see that once again, from a rolled ankle to a rehab center, alcohol had derailed my attempts to achieve at the highest level. The idea made sense, though, as I could be supported by my family and friends during the difficult time of early recovery, and besides, I was running out of options. So, I swallowed what was left of my pride and made the call.

I spoke with the hospital CMO, Dr. Charles Hedde, on the phone, and he invited me to come down for the day. Dr. Hedde was an incredibly kind and distinguished man, and I had always held a high opinion of him, even early in my youth. He was a compassionate and caring physician with a sincerity about his support for me and my recovery. I spent the day touring the hospital, met with the practice group, and reconnected with old friends who were all surprised to see that I was considering a temporary job back in my small hometown after spending the last twelve years traveling the country for school and training.

Throughout the visit I avoided the pointed questions and left a lot of things unsaid, since I was embarrassed by the truth behind this crossroads in my life. However, the visit went well, and after our meeting Dr. Hedde invited me to apply for a general pediatrics position and we began the process.

A few days later, his assistant called me to ask if I could meet with Dr. Hedde again, an unusual request given that his office was a two-and-a-half-hour drive from my home. I immediately knew that the same broken record of rejection was about to play again.

I agreed, I drove, and I was rejected again.

I was told the reason was related to insurance malpractice coverage, as there was a high-risk and low-reward benefit ratio in employing someone with a history of addiction for only a very short amount of time. It was not Dr. Hedde's fault; he didn't have a say in it at all. He was dignified, honest, and direct in his communication. He wanted to grant me the respect of telling me face-to-face, to apologize, and to add that he was proud of me. He told me that he would always be in my corner rooting for me, and that if I ever needed anything to please call him. For years afterward, he always made a point to check on me, and I will never forget that about him.

It is emotional for me to remember Dr. Hedde now. While still in the prime of his life, suddenly and unexpectedly, he passed away a few years ago after an abrupt diagnosis of cancer. His death left a huge void in my hometown, and in the hearts of his family and friends. I owe him a huge debt of gratitude for his kindness, love, and support during my recovery, and I never got the opportunity to tell him how much he meant to me.

After another heartbreaking rejection, I still had to move forward, and it seemed like all local options were exhausted. So, six days before Christmas, I took a job in Oklahoma. The position was as a general pediatrician and hospitalist on a Native American reservation in the southeastern part of the state. The convenient thing for me was that Native American reservations are considered federal land, therefore any active state medical license can be used to work on their grounds, and I didn't have to apply for an out-of-state license. It was a job, and they said yes, and I felt as though I didn't have any other choice.

I gave Lauren a kiss, packed the car, and drove the 735 miles in a single day, starting on the road a little after 5 a.m. The holidays are supposed to bring families together, but ours was seemingly being torn apart. It felt like I was chasing new problems by unsettling the foundation of my early recovery. But I had to work to support our family, and I had a long drive to think about how my career had gone off track.

Overnight, I went from three consecutive positions at highly reputable academic institutions to working in a newborn delivery nursery in a small town way off of the beaten path. Doing shifts from Christmas Day through New Year's would be a potent reminder that this was another holiday spent away from family, in tormented seclusion, to cope with my former transgressions on my own.

At least the drive down provided scenic vistas. The bluffs of western Arkansas, along the stone-carved route of Highway 49, contrasted with the worn-down gas station diner where I ate a rushed dinner before getting back on the road. I had managed to find one of the only smoking restaurants left in Arkansas, something I thought was illegal in most states in 2013. Taste is 90 percent smell, and a burger with a side of cigarette smoke didn't quite hit the Southern comfort food spot I'd hoped for on the trek.

Late in the evening, after almost fourteen consecutive hours on the road, I arrived in a sleepy, pasture–lined town. The sign read "Welcome to Talihina, Home of the Choctaw Medical Center. Population 1,099." The streets were pitch-black; a single row of storefronts and a solitary diner lined the main street, which sported one stoplight. As I drove past, I spotted a sign in the window of the diner that read, "Restaurant will be closed tomorrow due to family illness." A rodeo stadium was visible from the main drag. Off in the distance, I saw a sign pointing toward the medical center. I turned left out of the downtown instead, away from the hospital, toward a strip mall motel with a gravel driveway. Entering the parking lot, I saw one flickering street lamp, a row of twelve rooms, and a single mud flap-adorned pickup truck parked in the corner of the lot. A key had been left for me in a dusty mailbox with a handwritten note reading "Room 8. Enjoy your stay."

It felt like a scene out of a modern day Western—a quiet motel in a sprawling rural landscape, a horse pasture fence almost touching the bathroom window, a room dressed in '80s decor. As I brushed my teeth in the morning, I envisioned that old TV horse Mister Ed walking up to my bedroom window and eating an apple out of my hand. Reality was a little less sitcom-like. I quickly unpacked my car. I half-expected a flurry of cowboy hats, a showdown, and a final dramatic scene. Armed with a handful of dress shirts, my phone, and a rapidly sinking sense of self-worth, I felt like an inadequate dueling partner for the fight that was about to unfold.

Unsurprisingly, I was out the moment my head hit the pillow, having spent the entire day driving with only a handful of restroom breaks and coffee refills. The following morning, a new adventure was about to begin.

Driving into town only took a few minutes, as the entire landscape of the community covered only a handful of miles. En route to the hospital,

I passed a small white shack with aluminum siding and a neon "Liquor Store" sign that gave off a green glow. Beckoning a past version of myself, it planted a seed that began to grow as the weeks slowly passed by.

Talihina had all the trappings of a small town: one post office, gas station, a mom and pop grocery store, diner, and liquor store. Much to my excitement, a Subway sandwich shop had recently opened on the main strip, but if you visited after 12:30 p.m., the famous spread of choices were usually down to a single option.

I headed to the medical center and was pleasantly surprised at the scope of the facilities. The building was functionally beautiful, sitting right at the base of a pair of rolling hills in a wide-open meadow surrounded by cypress trees. On my initial tour, I saw a concrete helicopter pad carved off of the back of the parking lot, next to a white wooden cross draped in a wreath of flowers. Weeks later, I learned a helicopter had crashed in the field behind the hospital, claiming the life of a patient and injuring three of the other passengers.

The medical center was designed to serve all of the Choctaw Nation, so although it was situated in a small town, the facility served a large community that came from across all of Oklahoma, as well as the entire United States. In fact, a few weeks into the job, I treated a family that had driven almost twelve hours from Florida to get their annual medical screenings. I had the privilege of learning about their journey, while being confronted daily by the realities of an American culture that exiled indigenous people into disconnected boxes on a map.

Starting in this position was deeply humbling; I felt as though doing this work was beneath my training and skills. I felt like damaged goods, exiled to the hinterlands of modern medicine to pay a penance. For a decade, I had chased academic titles, attended prestigious universities, secured research grants, and authored publications in all of the celebrated corners of academic medicine. Having trained at some of the most respected institutions in the country had validated me. I sat on medical roundtables with graduates from Harvard, Stanford, and Yale, and for deep-seated reasons relating to my personal sense of inferiority, this all mattered to me. I was taught to value high achievement, and the scrawny inner child in me desperately wanted to prove that I wasn't some helpless kid from the middle of nowhere. Deep within, I held a constant fear of not amounting to anything and of being a nobody. I ran away from myself, out of the cornfield labyrinth of my youth, to bigger cities, fancier cars, and more exclusive destinations. And I didn't realize the guilt that would be attached to that upward mobility.

As I sat in the car outside the Choctaw medical center, I recalled the drive back into my hometown for the interview for the temporary hospital job, when I stopped at the local gas station and recognized a childhood acquaintance pumping gas into a beat-up truck. The rust on the undercarriage evidenced wear and tear from many miles driven down rutted country roads. The years seemed to have worn him down as well, and it made me feel a deep sense of personal conflict. I felt stuck between two worlds, lost between knowing who I used to be and searching for who I was trying to become. I wondered whether I should find a way to include the word "warsh" in a conversation, to summon the dialect of our youth, or mention my recent work on an esteemed hospital's stem cell transplant unit.

I put my head down, walked to my car, and didn't address him at all. Almost remorseful, I felt as though I had abandoned him, and myself. I was a refugee who escaped from a small town only to seek out a stereotypically superficial life. My entire family lives in that small town, too. I would come home for abbreviated visits and then immediately drive back out of their lives to chase my own selfish dreams.

In Oklahoma, forced to return to my humbler beginnings, I came face-to-face with the small-town boy who ran away from his roots—from the bullying, the disappointments, and the burdens of unrealistic expectations. I had purposely run away from him into a new and different life, and in doing so, I wanted to prove to myself that I mattered. But it never crossed my mind that I was constantly looking for validation in all the wrong places.

Far from prestigious universities where I had worked on cutting-edge therapies for neuroblastoma (a rare childhood cancer) just months before, the prairies of medical practice were an abrupt and humiliating recalibration. I would have been forced to swallow my pride if I had any left. But in this humble grounding, something started to change after I spent some time with my new boss, Dr. Marie Cole.

Dr. Cole is a kind woman, independent, soft-spoken, and hardworking. She and her husband ran a functioning ranch full time, in the hours before and after hospital work. On one of the first days she invited me into her office, but we didn't speak much about why I had landed in Talihina—she tacitly gave me permission to skip that part. I was there because I was a depressed alcoholic and couldn't get a job anywhere else, and on the inside I felt it every day. Dr. Cole didn't seem to care, though in a good way; she graciously stated in her opening comments, "Listen, we all have our own stories that led us here."

I immediately felt at ease and knew she would be a supportive colleague, as she seemed thrilled to have an East Coast-trained physician helping out for a few months. From the first day, she welcomed me into her work community with open arms.

So there I was, a trained pediatric oncologist now working in a small town, but maybe it was fate that I was assigned there, because only a few short weeks into the job a young patient walked through the pediatric office doors, bringing with her a new perspective.

Her name was Alex. Only a few days before our paths crossed, she had celebrated her ninth birthday at her family's local ranch, with pony rides, balloon animals, and a game of horseshoes. Her front yard brimmed with a loved-filled, exuberant celebration. A fragment of time later, she limped gingerly through the pediatric clinic front doors, and then collapsed on the waiting room floor. She was tall for her age, with long, fine hair down to the middle of her back. Her height made the fall seem more damning, as she lay for seconds that felt like minutes near the entryway door. Once her family ran to her side, she began to gather her senses, and the nurses ushered her to a triage room.

I rushed into the room, along with several colleagues. Her skin was translucently pale, and her parents noted a progressive weakness that had worsened during the past few days. As I talked to her, she moaned that all of her bones ached from head to toe. From across the exam room, the scattered bruises were readily apparent, covering every inch of her slender frame. As we stood over her, the thermometer registered 104.3 degrees, and I saw beads of sweat roll off the corners of her brow. We placed an IV line, blood was immediately drawn, and the medical team hounded the lab technicians for the results while they administered IV fluids.

When the results came back, her blood levels were incredibly abnormal: low platelets, low hemoglobin, and a markedly elevated white blood cell count with many abnormal cells. All concerning signs of a serious underlying condition.

In a surreal moment of self-importance, I showed myself into the hospital lab. From the glances of the laboratory staff, it seemed that physicians here didn't normally visit to look at their own microscope slides, but that was routine in my years of hematology/oncology training. I pulled out the chair, adjusted the lens, and quickly realized the diagnosis. This once-vibrant nine-year-old girl had fallen ill with acute lymphoblastic leukemia, and we needed to set up a transfer to Oklahoma University Medical Center to initiate further testing and treatment. I had trained for these specific moments of making this diagnosis, breaking the tragic news to the family and sitting with them during moments of shock and sadness. I was a pediatric oncologist fatefully assigned to be there for this young child in the middle of a small town on a Native American reservation in Oklahoma, and maybe it would help save her life.

After she was packed away in an ambulance and we said our goodbyes, the medical team huddled to support one another. We hugged, we listened, and we shared the moment. For the first time in my career, I felt loved and supported in a space where it felt safe to share the emotional difficulty of seeing a child dangerously close to death. It was clear that childhood cancer was not something that normally walked into the pediatrics office in this small town, and the moment affected everyone, so it was natural to share in those feelings. Our team bonded during the experience, the healing flowed bidirectionally, and it all meant something deeper. I felt honored to work alongside such compassionate and supportive colleagues. They appreciated my expertise, but more importantly, they accepted me for simply being me. For the first time in a long time, in the simplicity of those moments, I heard a faint whisper of the humanity of medicine calling out to me.

I spent most days working in an outpatient pediatric clinic, seeing children coming in for sick visits—mostly common colds, rashes, and ear infections—and then spending the afternoon checking in on newborn babies in the hospital. The work was relatively easy and relaxed, without the pressures and expectations of a large academic hospital. I caught glimpses again of the true heart of healing, and the real reason I wanted to work in medicine in the first place—to be of service to other people. I felt honored to work with an underserved population while gaining an education on the healthcare plights of the Choctaw people. I loved being of service in this way, but I couldn't just change a decade of personal and professional beliefs overnight. Over and over, I learned that biography mattered more than bliss.

So, after a relatively calm afternoon, I drove back to the motel, started to heat up an evening meal in the microwave, and heard my phone buzzing. I didn't answer, as the call came from a blocked number. (I'm an avoidant kind of person that way.)

On the voicemail was a woman's voice, sounding rehearsed in its cheeriness. "Hey, friend, just calling to check in. I've been thinking about you down in Oklahoma. I hope you are doing okay. But I wanted to let you know the paper I wrote got accepted for publication. Let me know when you get a chance to read it."

The voice was that of a colleague, an old friend, and for me it was an acute reminder. The message went on, but in my embarrassment I didn't want to hear it. Her thoughtfulness in reaching out felt like a needling. I didn't want anyone to know just how far I had fallen.

She could have said all the right things, but the blocked hospital number immediately reminded me that she was calling from the same esteemed hallways from which I had just been rejected in disgrace. I couldn't help but be reminded that the measures of success in medicine are tied to prestigious academic achievement.

I continued to let other people define what constituted success and failure for me, and after several weeks of wrestling with "how my career went off track," the demons of my past life came calling again.

I was bored and lonely; I would work from 8 a.m. to 5 p.m. and then go back to the motel room, lie on an unforgiving spring mattress, and watch streaming episodes of *The Walking Dead* on an iPad, when the Wi-Fi signal would allow it. The show felt like a metaphor for the life I was living: at the end of the world, aimlessly existing moment to moment in a survival mode, the zombies of active addiction lurking and waiting for a chance to resurface. All of the walls I had built during early recovery were shaking like a battered chain-link fence, barely holding back a relentless force.

Now isolated from my support network, I spent moment to moment white-knuckling my way through alcoholism recovery. It was clear that I wasn't doing what I needed to do to take care of myself, and eventually the neon sign lit up with a siren call back into the recesses of active addiction.

On a Friday night a few months after starting the position, I relapsed on a six-pack of beer. In an irrational justification, I had convinced myself that drinking beer would not be the same level of relapse as drinking vodka. I was ignoring what I knew about addiction, and creating a false hierarchy to comfort myself in my affliction. I was almost proud of this decision, as though I had made a wise choice, and convinced myself

I could move forward knowing I did not relapse on the same intoxicant that caused the initial calamity in my life.

In the end, though, it all seemed inevitable to me. I was off work for the weekend, and I spent my time watching Netflix and drinking at night while lying around the motel room. The tricky part of the equation was that I was mandated to submit tests into a portable breathalyzer four times per day. For medical professionals in addiction recovery, this mandate often extends for five to seven years after disclosure. So, I spent hours before the weekend calculating how much I could drink while still having my system clear before the 8 a.m. breathalyzer submission.

The ironic thing about having to use a breathalyzer four times a day to promote recovery is that when I wasn't even thinking about drinking, a blow into the machine was only four hours away to remind me I was an alcoholic. I could be mindfully consumed by the actions of a daily sobriety, yet have to sneak off to a workroom closet to secretively breathe into a device. With each forced exhalation, the shame cycle would begin again, in repetitive concentrated segments of time. I was always aware of the machine, as it literally hung over every breath I took for many years. On that night, I counted the minutes until the 8 p.m. breathalyzer test, after which I drank six beers within fifteen minutes, and then knew I had twelve hours for the alcohol to clear out of my system before morning.

I tormented myself for the entire weekend after that, wallowing in shame and guilt for the act of deceit. I spent the weekend chasing my own emotional tail, cycling between intoxicated relief and deep feelings of regret. I pictured the despair on Lauren's face as I sat in a green-tiled motel bathtub. In the finite, enclosed space of the tub, I buried my head under the water. With each submersion, the water level rose and the distance from my face to the surface seemingly deepened. In the moment, I didn't know how far down I had sunk, but I intimately knew what drowning felt like.

In a tunnel-vision flashback, I recalled lying on a street while grasping an injured ankle, feeling as though I had let down everyone who once believed in me—all for the comfort of another drink. I knew the path

I was headed back down, and that I couldn't sustain it again, so at the end of the weekend I called my recovery team in Indiana to disclose the relapse, and they encouraged me to come back home.

On a Monday morning, I let Dr. Cole know that I had to get back into my recovery network, seek out some further assistance, and get my life back on track. It was as though she already knew, and, with her characteristic loving acceptance, she stated, "The door will always be open for you here if you wish to come back."

For a year and a half, I had felt only the disappointment of abruptly shutting doors, but she must have seen something more in me. For the first time in a long time, here was an open door, despite my faults and shortcomings, and it gave me hope that I was capable of great things still to come.

After arriving home, I spent a few days with Lauren, but the highway soon called again. I knew I had to do a lot of hard work on myself, but it felt different this time. I felt the powerful potential of being a healer again, a potential discovered in the simplicity of a stripped-down practice of medicine in a small town in the middle of America. I could feel a new hope for my own worth, infused by the loving generosity of colleagues I never thought I would know.

I spent the following six weeks in a partial-hospitalization recovery program for working professionals in Chicago, Illinois. Here was an opportunity to reframe the perspective of my life from the thirteenth floor with an inpatient hospital view. A few weeks into the program, I walked into an Alcoholics Anonymous meeting, grabbed a chair, and pulled it into the circle. In the neighboring chair was an older gentleman with a cane in his lap, a gray beard, and a depth of wisdom in his eyes.

He said, "Welcome! First meeting with us?"

"First time here," I replied.

"Well, keep coming back."

I had always heard this at meetings—a casual greeting delivered in a rehearsed tone—but I could sense a deeper authenticity in his gruff voice.

"How long have you been coming back?" I inquired.

"Forty-two years now. One day at a time," he said with striking humility. He then went on to say, "It's talking to people like you that keeps me sober, and for that I thank you."

I didn't know what to say; I was dumbfounded. I just nodded as the meeting opened with a call for introductions.

I was struggling to appreciate myself, and yet a stranger had shown an appreciation for me I felt I didn't deserve.

In moments like those, I felt a greater calling to be of service to other people, and realized that maybe I, too, could help others through my own sobriety. Out of this connection, a sense of gratitude and grace was reborn as I began to see value in recovery again. I felt a new fire within, rising from the smoldering ashes of a dormant sobriety.

I reflected about the opportunity in Oklahoma, how much I appreciated the people I was able to serve, the community of colleagues who genuinely cared about me, and the reframing of what practicing medicine could actually be. There seemed to be a greater meaning in finding this opportunity, as it offered a reset to a chaotic life that had spiraled out of control. Working there revealed the simple truth of what it means to be a healer and to be healed. There were fewer variables, fewer inflated expectations, more humanity and more heart to the caring process. I was granted an opportunity to make a clean start, to define my own measures of success, and quit feeling sorry for myself by simply doing the right thing.

After six weeks of intensive treatment, I went back to Oklahoma to finish what I had started, with a new perspective and a plan for greater success.

CHAPTER NINE

The Prodigal Son

After finishing up my assignment in Oklahoma, I came back with something to prove, a prodigal son returning home. Through some old connections, and a few concessions, I received the opportunity to train again at Indiana University Medical Center with a plan to complete a one-year fellowship in palliative medicine. My addiction history was open for a world of insurance carriers, policy makers, and hospital administrators to see. The colleagues who knew about my addiction acted afraid of me, as if my presumed fragility required delicate handling. One person told my wife that they were afraid to talk about going out for "happy hour" in front of me, because they didn't want to trigger a relapse. For the most part people had good intentions, but this secretive kid glove condescension only yielded power to the disease. And good intentions or not, when people treat you differently because of a disease, well, they still treat you differently.

Several meetings were held in quiet offices to determine my "fitness" to take on a new work endeavor. It didn't seem like a great sign that I had to meet with four different deans just for a one-year training position at the hospital. In any other scenario I doubt they would have even known who I was, but in this situation they all had their eyes on me. I had a history, I carried a label, and I couldn't hide it. Yet I approached each day as though it was my only opportunity to prove the doubters wrong, and

I knew that although I couldn't control what other people said or did, I could control how I reacted.

In the first few months back, I made several professional friends who were in their own recovery programs, and another with her own harrowing tale of working with a serious medical condition. She didn't know what hit her for weeks and then months, while she continued to work day after day through declining health. She was a tall, middle-aged woman, a diligent and hardworking colleague with a brisk walk that captured her work ethic. She never slowed down, always running toward the next professional obstacles and then effortlessly clearing them as she climbed up the rungs of accomplishment. Then she started to develop symptoms, mild at first but worthy of notice. In her daily routines, she started to feel more and more tired, with an odd sense of breathlessness during her normal hospital rounds.

Over the next few weeks she started to sleep longer, finding it hard to get out of bed in the morning, and eventually had trouble falling asleep at night too. But she continued to work as several more weeks went by, and then one day found herself slumped over a stairwell railing, catching her breath before walking over to see a patient. In the days before she was finally rushed to the emergency room, her ability to focus on tasks had slowly dissipated, like smoke rolling off a freshly extinguished flame. Her mental capacities seemed overridden by her body's insistence on alerting her that something was seriously wrong.

In the emergency room, blood tests were drawn, imaging studies were ordered, and the reason for her months of declining health became evident. Her hemoglobin level was 4.2 g/dL. Normal for her age would be 12–15 g/dL, so in effect she had been walking around for months with 30 percent of the oxygen-carrying blood volume needed to survive. Her symptoms and test results brought a diagnosis of anemia, and all of a sudden her declining energy level over the past couple months made perfect sense. The images on the radiologist's screen revealed the culprit: uterine fibroids. These are an overgrowth of tissue, usually benign in nature, but can present with severe complications such as bleeding, miscarriage, or loss of fertility. In her case, the tumors caused heavy menstrual bleeding, leading to a profound loss of blood over a period of several months. Most of the time fibroids can be managed with medications, but occasionally they require surgical removal, with a modest chance they could come back.

The medical team ordered a blood transfusion and she was started on iron-replacement therapy. An outpatient surgical consult was also scheduled to remove the fibroids to prevent any bleeding complications. After the interventions, she slowly started to feel better. A few weeks later the surgery was performed, and she successfully completed the procedure without any setbacks. It took another three or four weeks before she really felt "normal" again, but she boasted about her ability to return to work on post-op day number four. Doctors often pride themselves on having a workaholic carelessness for their own health.

Back in college, she had survived the "weed out" classes and become a strong candidate for medical school while battling for a place on the valedictorian's list. Every step of the way, she was told she had to be strong to make the next cut. This dogged perseverance would be required to cure disease and save lives. So, when cracks began to appear, she hid them away for as long as she could. She and I were no different in this practice, as we both lived with fear of being exposed as an impostor. Her wounds were visible, mine were more difficult to see, but in the same attempt at self-preservation, we both projected a bravado to show that we could still work while we were sick. Inside, though, we were both terrified of being singled out for our perceived weaknesses, worried the rest of the pack would decide to leave us behind.

When all was said and done, after having felt unwell for several months, she went through a six-week treatment process, and then smoothly transitioned back into a day-to-day routine.

I listened to her story over a morning cup of coffee, feeling simultaneously concerned about her health and grateful for her recovery. But as I walked away from our meeting to go to a mandated drug screen,

I also felt confused as to why she never had to publicly disclose her condition. Why didn't she have to have ultrasounds every six months to monitor the status of her potentially recurring disease? Why didn't she have to submit regular blood samples to check her hemoglobin levels? She simply walked away from the coffee break back into her hospital routine, while I had to meet with dean after dean to assess my ability to handle the duties of my employment.

After the drug screen and another mandatory meeting, I walked down a long tunnel of an administrative hall. The middle of the workday bustled with fresh-faced administrators who came straight out of business school into the evolving world of modern healthcare. As they bounded past, I stopped in my tracks in the middle of the crowded hall, my eyes fixated on a bulletin board photo of a young nurse smiling with a youthful eagerness. Surrounding the photo, pushpin anchors adorned the cork with makeshift streamers and speckles of silver confetti.

The banner proclaimed "From PICU patient to PICU nurse."

A paragraph beneath the photo described her brush with death as a teenager from a rare medical disease. The illness, and the loving care she received, inspired her to pursue a nursing career, and now a handful of years later, she was gifted the opportunity to give it all back as a bedside nurse.

At the bottom of the page, she wrote "I know what it's like to be critically sick, so I want to share my experience with other people."

Standing in the hall alone, I wondered what it feels like to overcome a debilitating illness and then be celebrated for the compassionate perspective a disease could inspire.

For the first few months I walked on eggshells, and never fully unpacked the box near my computer desk, much like I had once left my blue coat hanging on an isolated kindergarten hook, just waiting for a moment when I might be shoved back down to the floor. In childhood, I learned to keep an eye out for unexpected threats around every corner. In adulthood, these suspicions and insecurities were validated by a constant flurry of blindside punches. The haymakers came from my own addiction, bouts of depression, bad decisions, and the out-of-control ramifications that followed. I often hear people say these types of negative experiences are good for you—that all hardship makes you stronger. I think it is one thing to have intermittent exposure to fight-or-flight scenarios, escape, and then return safely to a calm emotional state; it is another thing altogether to live in that state of mind twenty-four hours a day, fearing the worst is about to happen, and it is necessary to be prepared at a moment's notice. I can tell you, that level of heightened emotional stress is depleting, exhausting, and counterproductive.

Every time the phone rang, I half expected to be summoned into a meeting for an unceremonious expulsion. I awaited blunt words and shattered dreams, over and over again. Yet as time went on, I came to welcome the nonurgent phone calls and the diminishing of the daily intrusions of "How are you *really* doing?" asked with a wink and a nod and an implicit suggestion that there was a high probability of something being seriously wrong.

I went on with my work, and tried to do the next right thing every day. I settled into a new role and started to trust the people around me again, but I still kept a healthy amount of weight on a trailing leg, ready for flight at a moment's notice.

Toward the end of my successful fellowship year, I was offered a position as a faculty physician in a growing pediatric palliative care program at the Riley Hospital for Children in Indianapolis. The next year became a whirlwind of learning the clinical practice and running the inpatient and outpatient palliative care services, while staying focused on one day at a time of recovery. During my second year on the faculty, I was invited to interview for the position of Associate Pediatric Residency Director, a promotion that would entail assisting in the oversight and education of resident pediatric physicians. I had a keen interest in helping young learners, and a secret mission to try prevent them from going down the same path as mine.

When I interviewed for the position, it felt like a long shot, but another opportunity like that would likely not open up for several years, so I pushed ahead with the process. In the months leading up to this opportunity, I had finally begun to shake off the shame of my past. So for the first time, on a small scale during the interview process, I decided to proactively share my mental health story in the recognition that my journey was my greatest strength, replacing self-talk of "suffers from addiction" with "empowered because of it." I explained the incredible gifts of perseverance, strength, and passion I had been given because of my disease. I shared a level of empathy and understanding about the mental health of our colleagues that others may only know from a distance, and that I have lived and learned and had the privilege to help countless other people on their own journeys with illness. Across the table, a colleague listened and actually seemed open to this perspective. The interviewer was Dr. Rushton, a seasoned faculty member and an athletic man who loved the outdoors. For over a decade, he has successfully run one of the largest pediatric residency departments in the country. I would find out months later that he lost a close friend to suicide earlier in his medical career, and his empathy for me made perfect sense once I learned about this loss. In those moments of honesty, I was able to make a connection by being authentic, owning my journey, and presenting the legacy of it before someone else could falsely fill in the blanks.

I got the job.

But what happened next was something I never wanted to imagine again.

A few months after I accepted the position, tragedy struck our work community when, out of the blue, a harrowing early-morning phone call from one of my colleagues changed everything.

"Adam, can you come to my office as soon as possible? Doc Will was found dead this morning."

Dr. William was a mentor to thousands during his career, a first-class clinician who was also a gifted educator, not to mention a guy with an ebullient personality. He was a family man, a good man, and the last person I would have expected to have suddenly died.

I bounded into the back stairwell, emerging on the fifth floor. The corridor was flooded with brilliant Indiana sunlight. It was the kind of sun that shines upon the cornfields in my rural Indiana hometown, nurturing rays that make the stalks rise and ripen before your very eyes. I paused, feeling the warmth radiating through the high windows. Between the pristine hospital floors and the dazzling early-summer light, the corridor seemed almost impossibly white and pure in stark contrast with the eye-opening sorrow about to be revealed.

I felt a cold tingle down my spine, knowing, superficially at least, that he was in good physical health. I had a sinking feeling that once again suicide had claimed one of our own, and it wasn't long before this devastating fact was confirmed. There was an awkward, stunned silence punctuated by sobs when Dr. Rushton announced the loss of the man who had been the first connection to this hospital for many of the young men and women in the room. All seventy-five people present had enjoyed heartfelt conversations with, cried to, been guided by, and aspired to be like him.

Dr. William was the fifth colleague I had lost to suicide in the course of my short career.

As we sought mutual solace in the crowded meeting space, several people recalled seeing Will just a few days before with a smile on his face and a kick in his step. Looks can be deceiving that way, sometimes intentionally so. Together, we grieved as the institution's leaders attempted to console us. Dozens of heads hung and tears were shed in a silent gathering of shattered hearts. We stayed in the room for an hour, maybe two. But the words we shared about the tragedy felt hollow, as permission had not yet been granted to discuss the true details of his death.

What else could we say?

Initially, we had to tiptoe around the truth by simply discussing it as a "tragic and unexpected passing." Several colleagues who knew

Dr. William well spent hours going through emails, phone calls, and messages they had exchanged with him over the days and weeks leading up to his death. Personally, I wondered if Will had felt the way that I did as a man broken and beaten down by the personal exhaustion of modern medicine. I wondered if he had struggled with depression for a long time. I searched for ways to find an explanation, not only for myself, but to offer to other people. I felt as though I had a unique perspective to appreciate the depths of his struggle, given my own experience with suicidal thoughts and plans. I will never know what his own struggles, thoughts, or feelings were, yet I felt I could relate. I could understand the depths of a broken soul that led to the rational conclusion of suicide being the only feasible plan of escape. While I searched for a reason to share these thoughts with my colleagues, I realized that very few actually knew the details of my own story at the time. Therefore, it wouldn't make sense to them how I could have insight into this taboo world of suicidal thoughts and plans.

In medical school we had lost a fellow student to suicide, and it was never spoken about in a public forum. A few years later, a resident at another local hospital died by suicide in the overnight call room. When his colleagues last saw him, he was prepping for surgery, and he simply never exited the changing room. A few years later, another physician I knew shot himself after a full-day shift at the hospital. A chilling message had been sent out to his colleagues beforehand: "Get my wife, don't let her come home." No other words, no other clarification. Minutes later, the police found him dead at his home.

I had a story to tell too, and it was way past time to tell it. I couldn't live in fear any longer. So, in the days following Dr. William's death, I realized it was time to take a stand not just for a few mentors in a closed-door interview, but on a larger scale. The fear of retribution for mental health treatment as a medical professional was valid. Just a few years earlier, I had been publicly shamed and exiled out of academic medicine, and lost several work opportunities because of the forced disclosure of my mental health needs. The system punished and labeled me an outsider for a decision that also happened to save my life. That dilemma, for lack of a better word, was insane, and it had the potential to get worse. A state legislature was making national news by proposing a website to publicly disclose the mental health records of all licensed medical professionals in the state under the guise of protecting patient safety. In the same time and space, I was ready to share my own truth. This modern-day Salem witch hunt had to stop. I learned in recovery that I needed to focus on doing the "next right thing," and I knew what that was. It was time to move us all out of the darkness into a new light.

In the middle of summer, a few months after Will's death, I got behind the lectern in the 200-seat, oak-paneled Riley Outpatient Center auditorium. The grand space was standing room only that morning. In the audience were Lauren, a few close friends, my colleagues, and some of the top leaders of the hospital system. After a brief introduction from a colleague, I clipped on a microphone, walked up to the podium, and took a deep breath. I welcomed the air deep into my lungs, breathing in an impending liberation that would shake off the constrictions of my life. I looked down at my shoes, thinking about all the steps and states where my journey had taken me. Several years of weary travel down an uncertain road had led me to this moment.

Looking up, I saw Lauren in the second row with a proud smile on her face. In the weeks of preparation for the talk, she was the one who continuously encouraged me to dig deeper and share more. She was the first person to believe in me when I proposed opening up our lives in this fashion. She told me repeatedly that I had a chance to change lives and inspire others. She always believed in me, and in us, and I wouldn't have survived without her.

When our eyes met before my first words were spoken, she mouthed "I love you," and then, "You got this."

No turning back now, I thought as I gave her a subtle nod.

Then I began to address the crowd, uncertain of whether I would hear crickets or applause when all was said and done.

I opened with "My name is Adam. I have a history of depression, and I am a recovering alcoholic." I didn't hold back. I shared the brutal truth, exposing a raw vulnerability that brought me to tears during the middle of the talk. I bled my soul for the world to see as I shared about sitting in the woods, the gun store parking lot, and severe drinking as I considered ending my own life. I spoke of the profound strain it had on my marriage, the fracturing of my identity, and the loss of purpose and meaning. I discussed the loneliness, the numbness, and the never-ending cycles of self-deprecation in what turned out to be a cathartic self-examination. I connected my story to the dark unspoken truths of our profession. I needed to call out the secrecy and the broken systems that deter good people from getting the help they need and deserve. I wanted to shine a light on these cultural failings so we could move forward in productive ways to curb the ongoing epidemic. I also hoped this truth would help my peers make sense out of the loss of Will, relieve any shame over their own struggles, and confront the national epidemic of suicide in medicine. I had lived through this agony, and I finally found my voice to say it.

It was a massive risk to open up with this level of vulnerability. Yet I had decided that I truly had nothing left to lose. I found peace, too, in knowing that if I was persecuted for speaking out, I would at least know I had done so to help people. I could not be quiet while another person died in suffering silence. And in living authentically every single day since that first talk, the rewards have far outweighed the risks.

After fighting for years, desperately searching for any form of acceptance, I learned that I had to accept myself first, and show this self-love, self-acceptance, and pride openly in an act of vulnerability to create a space for a greater acceptance. Two hundred people strong stood up and, for several minutes, cheered and clapped for healing, recovery, and the conviction that we can all win this fight together.

A seismic shift happened for me in that moment, as I shook off decades of personal doubt and self-loathing. It took years, but I had crawled out of the woods to a higher purpose of healing by shedding a cloak of shame. I had a lot more work to do on myself, I knew, and I would have to protect my own wellness with boundaries as I embraced the demands of a newly accessible vulnerability. Sharing my story was only the beginning of the next chapter in a lifelong learning process of living as a man with a history of depression, suicidal ideation, and addiction.

From my years of struggle, I learned a great deal about the barriers to successful mental health and addiction recovery. I also learned from an older gentleman with a cane across his lap at an Alcoholics Anonymous meeting that in order to support my own recovery, I have to give it away to others. As a medical professional, it is my responsibility to encourage people to get the help they need and deserve.

The remainder of this book explores the lessons I have learned on this journey in an effort to give them away to help other people. These lessons have promoted a compassion and empathy that I strive to apply as a physician every day. On a long walk out of the woods, I learned how to take care of myself, fight the stereotypes and stigma of mental health conditions, and spark honest conversations through the power of vulnerability. I now know I am not tarnished or broken; I am in the ongoing process of helping others, and being healed.

Yet long before this very public stance was possible, and before I could use it to take care of other people, I had to learn a new way to take care of myself.

Chapter Ten

Learning to Take Care of Myself

"Do you love yourself?"

The question came from the lips of a soft-spoken therapist named Anna, and she welcomed the long, deafening silence I gave in response.

She sat in a sofa chair, hands on her lap, left leg folded across her right knee. Off to the side, a dimly lit lamp and a copy of Ernest Hemingway's *The Sun Also Rises* sat on an end table. Only a few feet away, I tried to camouflage myself in the dark shade of a charcoal-colored couch.

"I don't know how to answer that question," I finally said.

And with that response, I answered her question.

"Okay, we'll come back to that one. Who are you?"

I grabbed a frilly tasseled pillow from the side of the couch, clutched it to my chest, and rested my bottom lip on the fringe.

"I guess I'm here to find out . . ."

Rocking out of the cushioned depths, she lifted herself into a forward position with her fingers intertwined. In miniature movements, she pulled her fingers apart, and tapped the tips together. She knew she had her work cut out for her and seemed to be plotting her next move.

I was only a few days sober, and that initial counseling session went on for almost ninety minutes, with gentle intrusions into the anxieties

I was hiding away. One thing became abundantly clear in the line of questioning: I needed to find ways to truly understand myself before the harder work could begin.

In our initial work, we focused mainly on an immediate action plan for moments of alcoholic temptation, while we continued to unpack the depths of an evolving depression and addiction. The steps were to:

1. Remove myself physically from the situation.
2. Practice deep breathing.
3. Call my AA sponsor.
4. Call a friend in recovery.
5. Go to a recovery meeting.
6. Call my father.
7. Take a five-minute time-out (no decisions could be made).
8. Call Lauren.

This was mainly an addiction crisis intervention plan, but I knew it was only a Band-Aid over deep lacerations—intimate wounds that would be uncovered in the years of therapy to come.

"Do you know what triggers your drinking?" Anna inquired. Then she sat back in her chair, patiently waiting for a response.

"I just needed a way to stop the pain."

I was not intentionally withholding, but in providing only vague answers, I slowly realized that I didn't really know who I had become.

Developing self-awareness was never really a focus of my formative years, in training or in life. In an emotional sense, my adolescence was delayed until graduating from the twenty-sixth grade. I never understood the impact of being mechanically channeled through college, medical school, residency, and fellowships without so much as a pause for self-reflection. I just did what I was expected to do at every step.

At the same time, Anna understood that developing self-awareness was only a small part of the battle, hence the reason she opened the session with a question about my love for myself. She knew awareness of my emotions was one thing, but feeling worthy of loving emotions was a different thing altogether.

"I wonder if you felt pressured to simply conform," Anna remarked.

"Partially, yes. But I also just believed the promise that if I survived the process, it would all be worth it."

I delayed gratification for decades while stunting my own personal growth and emotional maturation. I became very successful at compartmentalizing the different segments of my life into neat, two- or three-year windows of time, and then simply moving forward without processing what I had just experienced. My box-packing skills were particularly well honed when it came to grief, trauma, frustration, and self-doubt. As I moved from city to city, I could have filled up a U-Haul truck like a real-world game of Tetris with all the emotional baggage I collected through the years.

Professionalism, procedural skills, medical knowledge, and exams were emphasized in my education, but I never took a single test related to emotional wellness and growth. Often, I felt like an eighteen-year-old cycling through a professional world, even in my early thirties. And I didn't notice it until I was being churned out the back end, beaten and broken, with a suicidal plan.

"I wonder if you worried about not belonging," Anna said.

"I felt that way from very early on in life. I always felt like I was living two different lives."

Professionally, I was incredibly confident and competent, but personally I had very low self-awareness. When the white coat came off, I did not know who I was. This disconnect between professional and personal maturity created friction between the processing of information within the halls of the hospital and within the walls of my home. The stunted processing was only exacerbated by being surrounded by like-minded individuals with the same level of training and emotional maturity.

"And how did that make you feel?"

"Ill-equipped," I muttered.

Over the coming months, I needed to take a personal inventory and needs assessment to help reintroduce myself to myself. I realized that medicine had taught me that my needs mattered less than everyone else's because someone else was always sicker, with more acute needs than mine. I realized that we are indoctrinated into a system that functions on the belief that others' needs are the sole priority. I put my own needs on the back-burner, because that seemed to be what the profession required. And I had done this for so long, I forgot how to even assess my own needs at all.

Anna listened to my account, and then asked, "Do you remember a time when seeing a patient triggered thoughts of your own addiction?"

"Yes. His name was Antonio."

Antonio was only nineteen years old when he developed osteosarcoma, a cancer of the bone. He had the '90s grunge metal hairstyle, parted in the middle and tucked behind his ears. He often wore Nirvana T-shirts and spoke of the bands of my youth as icons of a forgotten time. He came off as bold, confident, and self-assured, but I sensed a more complicated dynamic inside. Fortunately, he had successfully completed chemotherapy and his cancer was in remission. Yet he struggled with depression and chemical coping mechanisms during the treatment. His medical treatments had alienated him from his peers and isolated him from any sense of normalcy. Months later, it was clear Antonio was still struggling, still drinking alcohol and smoking marijuana to cope, and then he disclosed that he was taking Ativan, a benzodiazepine used for nausea, to fall asleep. Obviously, these issues had to be addressed. He needed to seek further assistance and counseling. He was incredibly defensive, angry, and resentful, and he blamed everyone for his problems. I could have held up a mirror. I saw myself in another person sitting across the treatment table from me, because I knew those feelings all too well.

At the time, in the professional hierarchy of treatment, I did not really know what my role should be, but I wanted to hug him and say, "I really do understand what you're going through." I didn't, because I was at a different point in my own recovery back then, which is to say I wasn't ready to be vulnerable about those sorts of issues just yet.

Anna asked, "Why didn't you hug him?"

"In medical school, I was taught never to get too close to my patients," I said.

She knew I was being evasive, so she probed further. "You've told me that before, but why else did you not hug him?"

"Fine. Because I didn't feel comfortable enough in my own skin."

Anna said, "Remember, we all bring our own experiences to the table, and being faced with those emotions again allows an opportunity for us to grow."

The session ended, and I left her office marinating in that thought for some time, acknowledging that I still had a lot of healing to do.

Weeks went by, and then years, as session after session dove deeper into the emotional rigors of processing complex events related to mortality and guilt that I had buried deep down for over a decade.

Anna opened another session by asking, "What was another event that really triggered your emotions?"

A few years into my recovery, I met a remarkable little boy named Luke who at just three years old had a relapsed and progressive glioblastoma multiforme (GBM), a highly aggressive brain cancer that had no cure. He was a bright-eyed, inquisitive, kind soul. I sat with him and his family for about two hours, getting to know them, hearing their story, and learning about their beautiful son and the living hell the last several months had been. Luke's father was incredibly loving and supportive, and we shared a connection right away. Luke's mother cycled between burying her head in her hands and being reflectively tearful. Over time, I became amazed by her courage, heart, and strength.

It was a true honor to befriend their son and sit with them during such a difficult time, but reflecting on it now, all I can remember is that his mother kept saying, "But there is a chance we can cure this, right?"

Unfortunately, the body of medical knowledge to date dictated that the answer was no. I simply said, "I wish that were the case." We cried, talked, hugged, and formed a bond that lasts to this day. Even in the face of a life-limiting illness, we tried hard to help Luke live well for several months. He was mainly able to stay at home, was given trials of some additional cancer therapies to prolong his life, and was eventually enrolled in hospice. He truly lived during that time, thanks to the exceptional love and care of his family. I was invited into their home on two occasions, and had the privilege of pushing him in a makeshift swing the family had set up in their basement. Luke smiled and laughed as the swing swayed back and forth with the gentle guidance of my hand. By his side, push after push, I relished sharing his innocent joy.

A few weeks later, when the time came, they decided to take a Make-A-Wish trip, knowing he was likely in the last few weeks of his life. At Disney World, he rode rides, enjoyed the sunshine, and truly celebrated every minute he had.

I called to check in with them during the trip, and Luke's father greeted me pleasantly from their hotel room. But five minutes into the conversation I heard a scream in the background—a guttural desperation that almost shook the phone. It was Luke's mother wailing that something was terribly wrong. There in the hotel room, only a few hours after riding amusement park rides, Luke had stopped breathing in his mother's arms. As I clutched the phone, I felt every mile of distance between us. Overcome by shock, I spent the next forty-five minutes talking Luke's parents through the final minutes of their son's life. I truly loved this family, and I could feel the heartache pulsing through my hand as I held the phone. Yet instinct took over as I walked them through the steps of keeping him comfortable as a local hospice came out to assist them. Recalling it now, all I actually remember saying was, "I am here with you guys" and then sitting in long pauses of silence. After the hospice team arrived, I made sure they were in good hands and then said a final goodbye. It was the hardest moment I've ever experienced as a physician.

How was I supposed to go home after something like that?

I walked to my car, past most of the staff in our office, and let out a primal cry. I was grateful that I was able to be there for them, and walk them through those moments of tragedy, but at the same time I was utterly heartbroken and shaken.

This loss felt different from the others I had witnessed. I tried to figure out why on the drive home, though I came up empty as to how it shook me so deeply. I pulled into the driveway and opened the garage door, now calmed down and ready to enter my home. I took one step in the door, and there it was right in front of me.

Luke was the first patient I had lost since becoming a father myself. At the door, a beautiful, curious, bright-eyed baby boy called to me from his mother's arms. I reached out for him, held him, and fell to my knees. I hugged him like I had never hugged anything before in my life as tears streamed down my face. I cannot imagine what Lauren was thinking in that moment, but she graciously stood there with us. I realized how much my identifying with this family stemmed from my love for my own son. I felt confused by the injustice of it all, and by the selfish gratitude I felt to be able to hold my baby boy.

To this day, Luke's family and I stay in touch. In fact, I had lunch with Luke's father in the midst of writing this book. We talked about our jobs, our families, and of course his beautiful son. At the end of the meal, he thanked me for giving them the gift of presence on the phone that painful evening.

"We couldn't have gotten through it without you," he said.

For months, I questioned every single thing I did in those heightened moments. I didn't feel like I had done enough. But the way he tells it, I couldn't have possibly done anything more.

Anna asked, "What feelings does telling that story bring up for you?"

"Sorrow. Anger. Peace. Heartache. Gratitude, to name a few."

"A lot of complex emotions," she said. "But what an incredible gift to walk with that family on their journey. What did you learn about yourself in the process?"

"Well, for several weeks I struggled, but you helped me see there are two paths forward."

The first path was to distance myself from experiences like these and guard my heart. But I knew this would lead to apathy for those suffering around me. Every day, I notice that this is the path most commonly chosen in medicine.

The second path is one of self-discovery, of self-awareness, and of processing emotion that can open up experiences of gratitude and grace in your life and forever change you by the act of leaning into them. The second path is to truly feel the emotions, connect them to your own human story, explore the reasons for their salience, and grow by engaging them. Only by developing self-awareness did I even begin to understand the power of this idea. I realized I can have an incredible impact by helping people during their time of greatest need. Luke and his family taught me how to live better and appreciate every day, to be present with people in the face of utter devastation and unspeakable sadness, and then to be able to kiss my son at night, whisper how much I love him, and knowing how grateful I am for each day with him, to truly, to my core, mean it.

"That is really powerful, Adam. But what were you telling yourself every morning when you woke up?"

"That I was worthless. *I wonder what I'll screw up today*—that was my first thought."

"Do you see the disconnect?"

For the longest time, I didn't realize I was my own worst critic. The narrator in my head had a fatalistic tone, like the film *Leaving Las Vegas*, in which the main character is in a hopeless struggle with addiction and thoughts of suicide. I was barraged by feelings of self-doubt, self-criticism, regret, shame, and unworthiness.

During the darkest depths of my depression, even my conscious mind quit caring enough to try to help me move forward; instead it just kept repeating one-word statements such as "bad," "worthless," or "weak." Even in the triumphs of initial recovery, my self-talk remained quite negative, often abetted by recurring themes left over from a past life. Even certain places, smells, or sounds would trigger thoughts like, *Nobody really cares about you.* Then I would find myself questioning my progress.

"Did you believe it?" Anna asked.

"At the time, there wasn't a doubt in my mind," I answered.

For years, I existed in a cycle of self-doubt and critical self-messaging. I remembered how once, a few weeks before the current session, I had felt completely off, waking up on the wrong side of the bed. The morning self-talk revolved around *I have to do this* and *I still need to do that*, which set rigid expectations for the day. I was wishing, wanting, and needing trivial things, and when I did not achieve them, I felt uneasy, as if the day was a waste.

"What can we do to break the cycle? Let's put together a plan," Anna proposed.

A few days later, I had a similar day of setting unrealistic expectations. Aware of how self-talk had started the day, I decided to make an action plan in the evening. So, that night when I went home, I left a note on my bedside dresser. The following morning, I woke up and there was the note. It said, "Today, I am grateful, I am thankful, and I am alive." This simple note allowed me to rehearse the monologue in my head and set a tone for self-talk for the remainder of the day. The tone was one of gratitude, of remembering to give thanks for the blessings in my life, and was a reminder that I had the privilege of living another day. On the surface, that next day went by just like any other, but it felt different—it felt paced, controlled, and appreciated. I took the day as it came, gave thanks for my experiences in it, and was able to build upon the morning's positive self-talk throughout the day.

After a few more months of sessions, Anna asked the question again: "Do you love yourself?"

"I've been working hard on it," I replied.

I was a little more prepared the second time around; at least, I had been working on it.

I realized that to love myself, I needed to be self-compassionate. I needed to create spaces that would allow for mistakes, setbacks, and failures, and to view them as opportunities to grow. I learned that the art of self-compassion is in discovering how to love yourself for being beautifully unique as well as perfectly flawed. I learned to see the good in all the things the world told me were different. I learned to own the truest forms of myself, and even allow them to flourish, while finding ways to avoid blame, regret, and cycles of shame. In the most basic terms, it was about finding ways to be kind to myself, and to prove my own worth through outward acts of kindness and acceptance. Over time, it became easier to love myself at home, but Anna knew that I continued to struggle within the culture of medicine, so she asked the obvious question.

"What about loving yourself while you're at work?"

"It's getting a little easier over time," I said.

The problem is that practicing self-compassion has become increasingly difficult. In medicine, social and cultural expectations are set to dangerously high levels. Social and cultural pressures require perfection 100 percent of the time—not only in technical practice, but also in outcomes and cures. The cultural standard is that individuals come to the hospital to get well, and any other outcome is a failure. We shamelessly promote the medical-industrial complex to combat death and dying. Culturally, how could we possibly expect medical professionals to grow in self-compassion, and to learn from failure, when perfection is always expected?

Built into the very fabric and framework of our system are mortality numbers, clinical outcomes, adverse event reports, and time since the last hospital-acquired case of pneumonia—all metrics designed to measure the quality of patient care, which affects ratings and the potential for hospital reimbursements by insurance companies. We have built systems that equate these metrics with clinical success, and it has had devastating effects on the mental health of the workforce. I remarked to Anna that in a lot of hospital systems, the sadistic moniker "harm report" is used to characterize adverse events that happen in the hospital setting. I lectured her on how the word "harm" implies a deliberate act, thereby placing blame directly on the institution and, more specifically, on the individuals providing patient care.

A patient fell out of their bed—harm report.

A case of hospital-acquired pneumonia—harm report.

An infection in an IV line—harm report.

Personally, I have never witnessed an "intentional act" of harm being done to a patient. I know it happens, but I have never seen it. Yet this language perpetuates a people-versus-policy dichotomy while executing a harsh judgment on what is likely an unintentional or accidental event. This choice of language does not invite a voluntary reporting of mistakes; it promotes secrecy, hesitancy, and animosity toward the system. It is the complete opposite of compassion and trust—using language to ascribe intentionality and/or malice to such events. The report is filed and the harm to the workforce is already done.

"And how does that make you feel?" Anna inquired.

"Angry that the system seems binary: perfection or failure. And it only seems to be getting worse."

As time has progressed, technological and scientific advancements have put more and more pressure on the individual providing care. Extracorporeal membrane oxygenation (ECMO) circuits, technology-guided surgical interventions, ventilators, new antibiotic therapies, drugs, and cures—they all add to the pressure. For with each new tool, procedure, medication, and intervention comes the loss of our ability to accept the uncontrollable. According to contemporary expectations, every broken piece of the human condition has a potential fix, and the expectation to find it is impossibly high.

The value of each "breakthrough" intervention is framed in monetary terms, but the underlying cost is much steeper when you factor in the new frame of mind it puts society in.

In a disease-based model of medicine, disorders of every organ system can be addressed with reasonable treatments to prolong life. So, when we inevitably fall short of achieving immortal solutions, a paradigm of failure, blame, and responsibility takes over. More and more, we live in a culture permeated by malpractice litigation and legal finger-pointing at a system expected to achieve immortal, controlled outcomes in a chaotic, uncontrolled world.

"I can see that. How does this affect you on a daily basis?" Anna asked.

"It is depressing, because I see the toll it takes on me and my colleagues."

I recalled sitting in a debriefing session with a group of young doctors, one of whom was in the corner of the room, head in hands and feet askew. He tearfully recalled attempting cardiopulmonary resuscitation (CPR) on a young girl with end-stage renal disease (ESRD) and multisystem organ failure. Simply put, the patient's kidneys and several other organs were failing, and she did not survive.

The next words out of the doctor's mouth during this session were "We failed her, I failed her. We didn't do enough."

The medical care in this case was diligent and exceptional clinical work. The patient had a progressive disease that worsened over the course of many months, leading to weeks in the ICU. The truth was, modern medicine had helped this young lady survive eight additional years. Yet here we were, sitting in a quiet room, discussing her physician's guilt for not saving her life. The expectation was one of perfection, of cure, without allowing for honest perspectives on mortality or the acknowledgment of years of incredible work that extended this young woman's life. I don't want to pretend death is not sad; of course it is heartbreaking. However, it was also not our fault.

This is what happens when we automatically equate survival outcomes with clinical performance; the results trickle into personal value, meaning, and identity. A personal void is filled with feelings of failure, regret, shame, and self-doubt. When medical practitioners are repeatedly bludgeoned by these events, apathy and depersonalization emerge as shields for self-preservation. An identity crisis may occur, since personal expectations are being dictated by unrealistic cultural ones. And what you have is a systematic failure of self-compassion.

"So, what can you do about that?" Anna asked.

"Well, I try to share about my own spiral down that pathway, as the end result of that line of thinking," I replied.

Feelings of failure can be controlled by redefining success, so I've learned to make my own standards that are consistent with my core values, rather than other people's expectations. In redefining success, my mantra has become: "There is a lot of pain and suffering in the world that I did not cause. All I can do is stand up to it and do my best to make a difference."

The power of this mantra is that it allows me to embrace the impact I can have in other people's lives, while also acknowledging that there are limits to what I can do. By adopting an external locus of control for certain aspects of my work, I can appreciate even the small interventions I can make to help people, and view those efforts as giant successes.

Anna said, "Sounds like you've set your own healthy boundaries and limits."

"Yes. I know I can have a positive impact on the world, but I can't fix things that are beyond my control," I replied. "With this philosophy, I can leave the unfixed parts of my work behind when I step back into my home."

Boundaries help me to draw concrete demarcations between the walls of the hospital and the walls of our home. For example, I make it the highest priority of my life to come home for dinner every night. I cook and then eat dinner with my family because I assign it the highest level of personal value. Before dinner, I take a hot shower or a hot bath, a calming exercise that allows me to wash away the day and reset myself for the evening with my wife and kids. In a Superman-in-a-phone-booth moment, I can walk into the shower a physician and walk out a father and husband. In the morning, I do the same thing before walking into work, pausing for thirty seconds outside the hospital to take three deep, resetting breaths that center me for the work to come. I also took the email off my phone, and I communicate clearly to my colleagues what I expect from them and what they can expect from me. Maintaining healthy boundaries has helped reveal my priorities and protect what matters most to my core identity, because I don't intend to lose that again.

Anna asked, "How does that make you feel?"

"Grateful that I have found plans that work for me."

In recovery groups, and working with Anna, I learned to welcome gratitude into my life. For many years, I had existed as a product of a medical system and never stopped to appreciate all the incredible blessings in my life. Even the small things, such as the flower beds outside the hospital that I walked past every day, or the dappled shade of the apple trees lining the path to the clinic, call for reflection. This lesson was solidified when I was blessed to travel the world to work in different hospital systems. Over the years, I have spent time in Mexico, Belize, Tanzania, and Kenya, and I was overwhelmed by the grace and gratitude of each nation's people. Some areas had very little to offer in terms of basic needs, let alone comforts, and yet the majority of the individuals I worked with were grateful for what they had, took stock of them on a daily basis, and were living genuine, happy lives. Those experiences opened my eyes to a worldview that challenged my previous belief system.

Anna asked, "What changed for you?"

Thinking deeply, I replied, "Well, in moments of deep depression, I was unable to see the other side of the coin; every flip inevitability landed on the wrong side. Now, I appreciate being able to flip the coin at all."

I consciously began to seek even the smallest things to be grateful for, minute by minute and hour by hour. Being in a recovery community, and reframing a world of experiences, showed me how much I already have to be grateful for, and that gratitude is found not in the spectacular, but in the ordinary and overlooked. People, moments, and places I had taken for granted for too long became some of the greatest treasures of my life. All of these things were spectacular all along; I had simply lost sight of them.

Once I came to recognize the blessings in my own life, I began to dedicate time on a daily basis to writing and speaking of my gratitude. This effort evolved over time into keeping a gratitude list. It started with a handful of items and has grown over the course of several years into a list with hundreds of entries, my wife, son, daughter, parents, sister, friends, and extended family serving as the starting point. A warm meal, a roof over my head at night, and not too much further down the list, Butler University basketball are also there. As the list has grown, it has come to remind me of a book I read in high school, *14,000 Things to Be Happy About*, by Barbara Ann Kipfer. As in that book, some of my entries are silly and funny, but all hold a significant value and meaning in my life.

The search has been remarkably powerful in itself, and the moments of reflection are priceless. There are many days when I find myself overwhelmed, defeated, exhausted, or short with my emotions. Taking a few minutes to ponder my list is immediately grounding, as I can center myself again and move forward with a little more patience and grace. I can give thanks for today and for the people, places, and things around me, and be instantly reminded of the greater fortunes of life.

"What happens when that doesn't work?" Anna inquired.

"Well, I have to use radical acceptance or distress tolerance to survive those moments."

In the sessions to come, I relayed examples of my practicing radical acceptance and distress tolerance in my daily life. When a colleague confronted me in an accusatory tone, I merely listened despite a boiling anger rising deep inside. In my years of addiction, I used alcohol to numb me to that sort of intensity, but in recovery I had to find a better way. So, I remembered that "this too shall pass," and that I cannot change what other people say or do, only how I react to it. At the end of her rant, she thanked me for listening, and I thought, "I didn't even have to say a word, I just stood there and listened—and it worked," which was strikingly better than previous such encounters when I would have spouted off and given the other person a piece of my mind. Then I would have replayed the moment in my head for days or weeks, letting the negativity live in my brain until it was terribly exhausting.

Over time I began using additional techniques, such as mindfulness, meditation, yoga, music therapy, aromatherapy, acupuncture, and writing. I started to pay close attention to my sleep, exercise habits, diet, and overall physical well-being. I expanded my toolbox to supplement the work I was doing in counseling sessions, but I also realized there was another role I needed to play. I understood that recovery does not happen in a vacuum; there was a cultural context that had to be addressed as well. Self-care on its own seemed trivial unless I became part of a greater revolution to influence society at large by addressing cultural and systemic barriers preventing individuals from pursuing better mental health.

CHAPTER ELEVEN

Stereotyping and the Importance of Individual Stories

"That guy looks like a real alcoholic."

When I returned to work after completing an alcohol rehab program, those were some of the first words I heard in the hospital. A colleague was speaking about a patient's family member in a condescending assumption about the man's story.

The ensuing conversation turned into barbs of judgment and falsehoods in an all-out avalanche of narrative destruction. I heard contrived theories about the "real alcoholic" in his absence, questions about his ability to be a loving father, make rational decisions, and care for his family.

My ears burned in the presence of these characterizations, and my heart cringed at the stereotypical accusations lofted casually from person to person. After having been protected by a buffer of early recovery, an outside culture came crashing back into my life when I returned to work and began to understand the perceptions of recovery amongst those who have not lived it. My senses felt heightened to a crippling extreme, sensitized by a personal understanding of what it is like to live under the weight of a stigmatized role, with a new set of standards and rules. It was under this pressure that my new perspective was born, and with it came a painful awakening.

I was now labeled an "alcoholic," "mentally ill person," "impaired physician," and someone with "mental health problems." I retreated further into myself, knowing that I, too, could be consumed by a cold avalanche of judgment hurtling down a mountain of shifting characterizations.

What if they knew I was an addict?

What would they say about me?

For how long would I be called an "impaired physician?"

I always cringe at the phrase "impaired physician." It is commonly used by treatment programs, hospital policymakers, and licensing and credentialing agencies to describe physicians with addiction and/or other mental health conditions. On many forms, in many contexts, and in many conversations, I have been called an impaired physician. Impairment literally means "functionally defective" or "under the influence of alcohol or drugs." This label projects a stereotype onto a diverse population of individuals with different medical diagnoses, and the looseness with which it is applied in our workforce is appalling. I learned that there are sixty-one different billing codes for alcohol-related medical conditions, and none for "impairment." So, if we are going to bill for these medical conditions, then we need to treat them as such. Now sober, and still labeled as an impaired physician, I guess I am just functionally defective. Naturally, this kind of thinking is hardly a great way to boost the morale of a person rejoining the medical community.

Over and over again, I heard inflammatory, blind assumptions made about others by the people around me—coworkers, friends, and acquaintances I knew and who knew me.

A few more weeks went by after my return, and the cuts deepened as I heard about "addicts" not deserving the same medical treatment considerations as others. I overheard single-word labels being forced onto complex human beings. I witnessed storytelling exaggerations dreamed up to fit preconceptions for the convenient purpose of categorization, without any attention to the nuance necessary to actually understand the individual.

I heard these portraits being painted as the lives they slandered played out in real time. The assumptions being made conjured images of a disheveled person, an abusive spouse, or a miscreant walking the streets in search of the next "fix." I overheard talk of estranged families and failed rehabilitation, with the inevitable dramatic arc of living with homelessness. These were "socially acceptable" brushstrokes concocted to capture what is often misunderstood.

Naturally, I imagined the stories that would be told behind my back, as I recalled overhearing gossip and innuendo about other colleagues "losing their minds" and "spiraling out of control," and envisioned a person being an incoherent risk, slurring their speech and bumping clumsily into hospital walls. I pictured cinematic scenes of a young doctor reaching for the bottom drawer of his desk, hands shaking in an unsteady attempt to grasp another hidden-away drink. An ominous musical score would play as the drawer revealed empty bottle after empty bottle and the doctor fell to his knees, writhing on the office floor, a morally corrupt mind bemoaning his unfulfilled urges. In the past, I watched this movie from the proverbial balcony, with a somewhat detached curiosity about the plot. In recovery, I was in the front row, intensely focused on the doctor's pained expression, and hearing all the whispers from the audience behind me.

I imagined back-hall conversations about how I was a reckless deviant unfit to practice medicine. I conjured whispered speculations about how I was scamming patients for a bottle of their unfinished pills. And I had thoughts of people suggesting that I had snuck into a linen closet to consume another swig to survive the day without withdrawals. Gossipy insinuations that I was selfish, careless, and lacked concern for the well-being of the people in my care invaded my mind. I lived in stereotypical boxes with dotted-line connections to mug shots, court cases, and the evening news, while people's assumptions influenced their attitudes about "how to handle" unreliable and unprofessional individuals such as myself.

I saw how the story would be told because I lived it. I was labeled a "risk to public safety" after voluntarily disclosing my struggle and proactively seeking treatment and recovery. I was a black eye on the field of medicine, a risk that had to be mitigated, with a true story that mattered less than the narratives imposed to fit me into a gritty cultural box.

On tremulous shoulders, I carried the heavy labels of "alcoholic" and "impaired physician," and these words themselves wrote the rest of the story for public consumption. But the truth is that every person has a unique story, one deeper and richer than any preconception.

For years, the truth drifted further away in a hot-air balloon billowed into flight by the daily fuel of misguided assumptions. And the fall from that height inflicted deep personal scars on me, some of which I am still recovering from to this day.

The truth is that I was sick and I struggled, but I was afraid to reveal the reality of my affliction. I continued my duties as a physician, rarely missing a day of work, and yet my experience was colored by shades of gray. Some parts of the stereotype may actually be true, but the whole is greater than the sum of these parts. Depression is a disease, and addiction is too, but I also accept responsibility for my actions. I try hard every day to accept, own, and move forward from the behaviors of my past. I accept that I drank alcohol and got behind the wheel of a car more times than I want to remember. I acknowledge that I openly drank in the car, hid bottles underneath the seat, and broke numerous laws in the process. I acted selfishly time and time again. I made a lifetime's worth of mistakes in only a few short months. I piled bad decision upon bad decision and they accumulated into a mass of unending regret. I lied constantly and lived a secret life—cheating my friends and family along the way.

Alcohol changed me, and in all the wrong ways.

In this disease, I was deeply wounded, and tried harder and harder every day to hide it. But no matter the depths I fell to, I never became a disease. My life will always be more complex than a textbook medical diagnosis. So, I write this as a challenge to the status quo of how we in medicine treat each other in the daily practice of healing. As the medical culture continues to struggle to support its workforce, and with a wary, suspicious relationship between patients and the medical system, we must find a better way, because the current practice has set a negative tone for the people under our care.

One reason for this ongoing failure is that we continue to rely on stereotypes and a depersonalized funneling of individuals into a scientific approach that does not recognize our humanity. I was never more aware of this than when I walked into a new primary care doctor's office after a few years of recovery. I was handed a form on a clipboard with spaces to fill in: age, demographic, insurance information, four columns of medical history boxes to check yes or no on.

Fatigue?

Headache?

Nausea?

Loss of appetite?

Depression?

The list went on and on, and the message became abundantly clear. Patients are a collection of data points, and the form is an efficient substitute for the time we have stolen away from narrative medicine. More than that, the form is a manifestation of how we are instructed to practice medicine in the first place—that is, to ask pointed questions that elicit an inventory of symptoms, collect the symptoms into a list of potential diagnoses, and whittle down the list until a disease is identified.

After laboring through a few more columns of checked boxes, I looked down at my phone. The screen saver was a family photo of Lauren and our two children, a picture I had proudly shoved in the faces of captive colleagues during a work barbecue a few weeks earlier. I wished I could have translated the picture onto the form, and I hoped I would have the opportunity to describe my life in a richer language than yes or no.

Last year, I walked out of our outpatient clinic and across the medical campus, stopping as I passed the outpatient pediatric dialysis unit. I knew some of the patients fairly well, and a few others only from a distance. Distilled into the medical calculations, all the patients had a history of chronic renal failure, meaning their kidneys were no longer filtering blood at the appropriate levels, which can be a life-threatening condition. Renal failure is a broad category with a multitude of causes, some of them secondary to genetics, trauma, medication, infection, and/or coexisting medical conditions.

I stared into the unit, taking in the totality of the process unfolding before my eyes—a beautifully choreographed dance of humans and machines in a mechanical, box-step routine. From the outside, all the treatments looked the same, and all the diagnoses did too, with everyone huddled together in a single room, with defined stations and obligatory roles for the medical professionals. On the surface, a group of people were boiled down to a treatment algorithm, a flow diagram with one strategic plan, in the same prescribed space.

As I continued past the unit, I read a plaque on the wall that stated "Dialysis Unit: Dialysis Patients." My mind shuttled back to the time I played piano outside a locked steel door, wondering about the individuals that resided behind the deceptively simple sign.

At one point in my career, I, too, became calloused in accepting the stereotypical view of disease and diagnosis after grinding through education, training, and hours of emergency room shifts seeing one rash, one cold, and one abscess after another. After a few years of residency, I felt the cumulative effect, and it became easier to accept the minimal truth and move on to the next thing. Our medical system teaches and rewards this type of superficial efficiency. And then one Tuesday morning, I got a phone call.

"Adam, I need your help," a voice mumbled, desperately fighting back tears.

"What's wrong, Amanda?"

It was my sister, calling from the emergency department of our local hospital, the fast-paced buzzing of a busy waiting room echoing around her.

"Your niece just had a seizure," she said. "I'm scared and I don't know what to do." Her voice was cracking.

"It's okay. We'll figure this out together," I reassured her.

From our conversation, it became readily clear that my four-year-old niece Colette had suffered a febrile seizure along with a common-cold fever, and she was going to be just fine.

A simple febrile seizure, when not associated with atypical symptoms, is a relatively common diagnosis in children six months to five years of age. The only treatment is reassurance for the patient and the family. At a glance, the typical diagnosis is that this disease is benign—from a medically educated perspective, of minimal worry, with no need for intervention. But my sister is not the mother of a disease. Colette may have been fine, but Amanda surely was not.

It was humbling to remember that when it happened to my sister, this event was the worst hour of her entire life. She called me overwhelmed by fears that any mother would have after seeing her daughter shaking uncontrollably on the kitchen floor. Months later, Amanda woke in a feverish sweat from a nightmarish recollection of Colette's eyes rolling back in her head. For my sister, it had been a life-altering moment, one she will never forget, and I couldn't imagine the subsequent trials she had lived through. No matter how routine or superficially defined the diagnosis, for the impacted family or individual, a medical event may be cataclysmic. My sister's fears were not benign, and without love and kindness from a local nurse and her baby brother, those events could have left long-lasting scars.

I fully acknowledge that I sometimes fail too; I am not perfect in this practice. Not that long ago, our team was called to see a new patient, and I let my own stereotypic assumptions momentarily cloud the truth of the situation. The young man involved was a teenager with a diagnosis of spastic cerebral palsy. He had been in the hospital for three or four weeks after a successful spinal-repair surgery for scoliosis. He had remained in the hospital recovering from the surgery, with some minor healing issues around the incision site. I walked into the room, immediately noting that no family members were present as a nurse and her assistant flushed his IV line. The young man was lying in bed, his head arched back, and he seemed to be staring at the wall. Instead of walking up and introducing myself, I went straight to the nurse and asked, "Is the family around today?"

She said, "No, but are you here to talk to Josh?"

With that, Josh turned his head and said, "Hi, how are you?"

In the first seconds of the encounter I had assumed Josh couldn't talk, and in doing so I failed Josh. A fair number of teenage patients with severe cerebral palsy are nonverbal, so I had guessed it would be difficult to talk to him, and failed miserably at introducing myself to boot. All of this happened within a ten- or fifteen-second period before I realized the fault in my ways.

I turned around and said, "Well, hello, Josh."

Josh went on to tell me about his hospital stay, that he attended a local high school, that he was in the tenth grade, and that he loved the Chicago Cubs. He was not staring at the wall; he was watching a baseball game on a television on the other side of a curtain. He grinned ear to ear as he told me about his favorite sports, his family, and how he couldn't wait to get back to school once all of this was over with. I was embarrassed by my own clouded judgment in that brief initial moment. And if I had not reset and humbly admitted my shortcomings, I might have missed out on getting to know a remarkable young man.

I share all of this to make a larger point, not because I think disease-based subspecialized medicine is bad or the model should be entirely changed. I make this assertion because we should not be surprised that we continue to stereotype people based on their disease. To practice evidence-based medicine in a disease-based model of healthcare is to group people into generalized types from which assumptions can be made, because reliable, reproducible scientific evidence relies on it. This is such a delicate tightrope to walk, because we also have to remind ourselves that an individual human being with unique life experiences resides within the constellation of his or her symptoms. The entirety of a human life will never fit into a diagnostic algorithm. The greatest impediment to providing good holistic care exists in this paradox of stereotyping by disease, and this practice encourages a neglect of our humanity.

A six-year-old girl in the ICU is not an upper GI bleed from acute liver failure. She is Katelyn and she loves stuffed animals, her baby brother, and dressing up like a princess. She loves her favorite pink blanket and watching cartoons.

Likewise, I am not a thirty-eight-year-old with a history of depression, alcoholism, and suicidal ideation. I am Adam. I love traveling, music, poetry, spending time with my family, and the Butler Bulldogs (and I also like stuffed animals). The evidence-based disease model fails to care about any of that; in fact, it works in contradiction to it. My uniqueness becomes a confounding variable that must be controlled, and my individuality must be randomized into nonexistence in order to yield reliable scientific results. These personal characteristics get in the way of data analysis and predictive value. The system runs efficiently for the purpose of technical medical progress and scientific advancement when all of these other characteristics are taken out of the equation. Thus, the practice that focuses on disease falls dramatically short in assessing the larger picture. This technical mind-set may yield progress in terms of treatment options, but it also sacrifices our ability to actually heal.

In reality, medical conditions do not show prejudice, and there is no stereotypical alcoholic, or stereotypical depressive.

I am one face of alcoholism.

I am one face of depression.

Josh is the face of one young man living with cerebral palsy, and Katelyn is the face of one young girl battling liver failure.

I have witnessed their brave responses to complex medical conditions, and I, too, have battled my own conditions. But without discrimination, we are all part of the same human condition.

I've sat in recovery meetings alongside individuals from every walk of life, without any sense of separation. Medical conditions, including mental health conditions, have no prejudice, and recovery from them should have no limitations. But part of that recovery should involve validating the lived experience of the individual, and remembering that it is a true privilege to be invited into another person's story. Now more than ever, I am aware that we are all perfectly imperfect human beings, trying our best in this world, and we all have unique stories to tell.

Combating these stereotypes takes time, effort, energy, and a willingness to open oneself up to another person's perspective. I share my own truth publicly to drown out the stereotypical prattle spewed during times when I am silent. And I listen to others' stories so their own remarkable truths are heard.

When Katelyn, my young patient who loved stuffed animals and princesses, started feeling better, she walked down the hall, across imaginary barriers, and shared her scary hospital story with a young boy recently diagnosed with leukemia. She just wanted to play. She did not know of the diagnosis assigned to her, of any stereotyping or expectations. She did not superficially judge the other children sharing the same hall; she only wanted to connect with them in a fundamental way. She did not know there was a box, or simply did not care. She reminds us that the goodness has always been there, in all of us. She just wanted to connect to another human being and share her story. In the corner of the hall, I was watching and listening to a better way forward for us all.

Chapter Twelve

Standing Up to Stigma

To keep my medical license, I was asked to write a letter to be published in a public newsletter, apologizing for my addiction.

The wheels of bureaucracy grind slowly, so more than a year after my voluntarily disclosed alcohol relapse in Oklahoma, a litigation process ensued. I owned a professional record devoid of malpractice claims, with no hospital-related or legal issues, and not a single patient complaint in over a decade of medical practice.

Shortly afterward, the phone calls from lawyers and investigators came, while a probe was opened up into the most intimate details of my life. I lived through a condescending line of questioning laden with doubt of every word I spoke, and an insistence on providing evidentiary proof that I, an "addict," could be believed. All of this was carried out to determine whether I should retain a professional medical license and continue to practice as a physician. In a criminalization of my medical condition, I was forced to hire my own attorney to fight the implied allegation that I was a morally corrupt, legally deviant doctor, and a "risk to public safety."

During the medical board hearing, I defended myself regarding the gaps in work history and the academic probation that had been assigned to me for being in a recovery program and taking thirty days away from medical practice for treatment. I was required to publish my medical history, for consumption by the public, so that I could continue to work in a field I had dedicated my life to.

On the day of the hearing, I arrived shortly before 9 a.m. to wait in a line of cases to be heard before the medical licensing board. I waited and I waited, with an anxiety culminating in bouts of stomach-turning nausea about the future of my life and career. In a public forum, I overheard private details of other people's lives being aired for all to hear, as a local news reporter took notes in a corner of the crowded basement room.

After waiting around until 4 p.m., I heard an assistant make an offhand comment from across the aisle: "Oh, the alcoholic case is up next."

Let the stone throwing begin.

As I walked up to the podium, I could sense silent heckles and snarls rising into a single-minded hysteria. In this public place, with sixty people present, a surreal moment of public branding was unfolding. The clear message was that I should be ashamed of my actions and needed to be punished. The board imposed a probationary status on my medical license and a monetary fine, and also demanded the publication of a letter of apology. Head down, I crawled away from the meeting, questioning why I had even disclosed my condition in the first place. I still bear the scars of this public wounding.

This is the face of stigma. But I would argue that it isn't just that; it is also discrimination. Employers are not allowed to ask individuals about their gender, sexual orientation, religion, ethnicity, or physical health. Yet medical licensing boards are still asking intrusive questions about individuals' mental health conditions, in a clear challenge to the principles of the Americans with Disabilities Act. This federal mandate seems to be conspicuously overlooked at the state and local medical licensing board level.

I knew I needed ongoing treatment and accountability, but those interventions can't be equated with punishment and public shaming. I was stereotyped as a deadbeat alcoholic in a narrative that spun out of control before I could even attempt to reel it back in. Stigma is a mark of disgrace and deviation from the cultural norm that gets superimposed over one's individuality. Because I dared to seek treatment for my medical condition, shame, judgment, and punishment followed.

In medicine, the greatest irony is that a majority of hospital systems tolerate rates of distress among their workforce of more than 50 percent. Physician suicide rates are significantly higher than the national average for all professions, and some of the highest rates of active, untreated mental health conditions occur among individuals working in medicine. I have to infer that this at least partly due to how we treat our own. Maybe what has been accepted as the cultural norm is unsound and needs to change. The reality is that, statistically speaking, the norm is to suffer as a medical professional, right alongside the patients. Unfortunately, the norm has also been a systemic indifference to this plight. Individuals like myself who live with these conditions are often left to feel different, afraid, guilty, and humiliated—if they're fortunate enough to survive at all.

In recovery, I witness the persistence of this stigma every single day with colleagues and patients. I was privileged to become close friends with a young physician who was also in a recovery program for depression and anxiety. She was a few years behind me in her journey, and I served a mentoring role on her path of self-discovery. One day she came to me, tearful and distraught, because she was given a hard time by colleagues who called her lazy and selfish for taking two days off from work. The others were forced to rearrange their schedules to accommodate hers. This is a difficult situation, especially in the context of other individuals feeling overworked and distressed as well, but in this instance the others were at least aware of her ongoing treatment.

Would they have said the same thing if she were in treatment to recover from a broken bone?

The whole weight of stigma as a cultural barrier comes into play in situations like these. The system we have built expects medical professionals to work even when sick, because someone else is always sicker. For the vulnerable individual seeking help, it feels unsafe to disclose personal struggles to colleagues, and the cultural expectations surrounding the decision to take care of oneself create feelings of guilt. In an often understaffed, under-resourced workforce, when one domino falls, the rest of the fragile infrastructure starts to crack as well. Exhausted, overworked, underappreciated colleagues mumble, "I should be the one who gets two days off," and perhaps justifiably so. When my young colleague returned to work, gossip and rumors spread like they might in a high school cafeteria.

Stigma is often used as passive permission to avoid deeper understanding, and to perpetuate feelings of disapproval for any deviance from the social norm. The social norm is that physicians come to work even when sick, and this norm was allegedly violated by my colleague, propagating feelings among her colleagues that principles of fairness had been subverted. The problem here is that the cultural norm itself is faulty. Given that more than 50 percent of the medical workforce is distressed, the cultural norm should be that we take care of each other when we are sick.

In my own medical institution, we combat stigma and take care of each other by normalizing the conversation around seeking treatment. For our medical residents, a few colleagues and I started a process of opt-out counseling by scheduling sessions for *everyone* in the medical training program. An individual can decline the appointment without any repercussion, but we value and protect the time for people to go to the sessions. Since the norm is that everyone is scheduled to go, no one feels different for seeking out and receiving this level of support. As a result, once secretive conversations about attending counseling now happen openly, and the physicians actually feel more comfortable going.

However, the stigma persists. After a recent lecture I gave, a student approached me to ask if we could talk in private. She shared that both of her parents were in addiction recovery, and her father had recently lost his job as a therapist because of it.

She cried and said that every day, in every rotation, her colleagues, mentors, and other professionals make insensitive, hurtful comments about "addicts." Coming to work on hospital rounds had become unbearable for her due to such stigmatizing and abrasive language. She would spend the weekend with her parents in acute recovery and feel as though she were living in a state of personal and professional shame. She wrestled with how to balance a façade of professionalism with an ongoing internal turmoil.

She expressed an unease about whom she could trust with this information and whom she could safely confide in about why she needed to leave work early on Fridays to participate in her father's family treatment program. She was struggling to find her voice and play her role on her medical team while wanting to stand up and shout at the top of her lungs. She wanted to unleash a guttural scream of advocacy in defense of those she loved most dearly. All I could do was listen, give her a hug, and let her know I stood with her. It reminded me that stigma fails to acknowledge the collateral damage of what people in recovery go through, and sometimes even fails to reveal who is really being hurt.

Shortly after this lecture, I read an article about the recent suicide of a medical student. I saw another example of the pervasive nature of the stigmatization of mental health conditions there on full display. Unfortunately, like mass shootings, medical student suicides are happening at a rate approaching a critical mass, numbing us to their gravity and drawing them away from newsworthiness. This particular story told of a young woman who jumped to her death from of an eighth-story window. The article went on to review her accomplishments and her relationships, much like an obituary. Then I saw a comment beneath the article from another medical professional.

I am sure it was intended as an expression of sympathy, but instead the comment graphically exposed the truth about how a lot of people view individuals with mental health conditions in our field. The commenter wrote, "We were all worried she was not strong enough to be a doctor."

After my initial shock and horror at reading such a thing about an individual who had just passed away, I collected myself and tried to process it.

Why was I even surprised?

This was probably the most truthful statement I had read in all my time experiencing and lecturing about mental health recovery. This was one person being honest about the culture we have created. Stigma declares that depression is a weakness, and strength and resiliency are prerequisites to protect against it.

My colleague Dr. Seagrams was diagnosed with breast cancer several years ago and took three months off to undergo treatment. She was successful in her initial therapy and remained in remission for about two years. She continued to work off and on during the next few years of her recovery, in a loving and supportive workplace now filled with pink ribbons, coworkers with shaved heads, and a break room stocked with snacks. A fundraising walk was organized on her behalf. After her long battle with the disease, the cancer returned and she lost her life to it, but she was a fighter and an inspiration. She was a hero and gave it everything she had. These are true statements about an amazing woman, but absent from the article reviewing her life was the statement, "She was not strong enough to beat her cancer."

Another colleague, Dr. Allen, was diagnosed with type 1 diabetes early in her career, and maintained an exceptional program of self-care. She was meticulous in her blood-sugar monitoring, and took pride in the work that she did to manage her disease. She would post online results from her lab reports, and tout the success she had controlling the disease.

The comments about her care regime proclaimed, "amazing work," "inspiring," and "tough as nails," all the way down her social media page. She was diligent in developing a medical plan that worked for her; therefore she was an incredible success. Nowhere on that page did it say, "You are a weaker physician because of your disease," or "You were not tough enough to cure your diabetes."

That last line may sound crass or comical, but when you extrapolate it to include the experience of individuals living with mental health conditions, it is an appalling reality. Rarely heard are statements such as "inspiring self-awareness." Instead there are offhand comments such as "lazy" or "weak," or descriptions of character flaws and a need for a thicker skin.

While it is considered a sign of weakness when a person is unable to overcome a mental health condition without outside resources or support, no one called Dr. Seagrams lazy when she took three months off from work for her treatments, and we are inspired by Dr. Allen's ability to focus on and execute a self-care plan for a disease that is not stigmatized.

The fact is that culturally, we view individuals with mental health and/or addiction conditions as flawed, broken, inferior, or weak. This stigma assigns a seat for us at the end of the table. Medicine is no different in this regard. It is astonishing that those of us actually treating individuals with these same conditions are not exercising the compassion needed to understand the harm it does to project a label of weakness onto other individuals. Viewing them or us as broken, flawed, and inferior reinforces a culture that does not permit changing seats at the table. These practices shame individuals into taking their assigned corner seat, fearful of seeking help and treatment that may actually save their lives. Stigma holds people down and actually works against the common medical knowledge that a lot of these conditions are treatable and not caused by character flaws.

Tragically, a lot of people suffering from mental health conditions already exist in self-deprecating cycles, while desperately seeking their own forms of affirmation. In the depths of my depression, I didn't feel worthy of a seat at the table at all. I stigmatized myself, too, as I regressed into a childhood state of isolation, my own sense of worth being directly linked to the actions and attitudes of those around me. From an early age, I lived with the self-defeating belief that I deserved to be bullied. I desperately sought affirmations from other people, and when I didn't find them, those absent affirmations morphed into cruel self-talk.

I am different from everybody else.

I should have done better.

I should be ashamed of myself.

In this cycle, I lived in a self-fulfilling prophecy of not feeling as though I was good enough, and then being told I was right about that all along. When I initially returned to work after rehabilitation treatment, a coworker who was returning from her maternity leave was greeted with balloons, hugs, and a celebration in a workplace meeting room. Colleagues clapped and cheered that a new life had been brought into the world. I sat quietly in my corner seat and almost chuckled, as my life had been brought back into the world too, but no one seemed to notice or care.

In sharing my story, I want other people to feel there is room at the table for their story too. I don't want them to feel as alone as I did in those initial years of recovery. I stand up for my colleagues so they can feel showered with balloons, hugs, and celebrations for reclaiming their lives. But I don't stand up just for them. I also won't stand silently by while patients, their friends, and their families continue to suffer from the deleterious effects of stigma.

Her name was Chloe. She was a single mother, and her daughter was critically ill in the intensive care unit. Her baby girl was born with a complex heart condition and clung to life after two major surgeries. In the surgical wing of the hospital, the baby was enveloped by a tangled web of wires and surrounded by an array of alarms and blinking lights.

In the middle of an otherwise ordinary day, an alarm sounded, echoing out into the hospital halls. The blaring alarm signaled that Chloe's only daughter, Alexis, was struggling to breathe while on her life-support machine. A flock of white coats crowded into the room in a flurry of action. In a corner sat Chloe, head in hands, caught in the depths of an uncertain fear I could never even begin to imagine.

Chloe's story was as complex as her daughter's heart we had once operated on, with enmeshed layers of life experiences. On the surface was a picture of a baby in a bed and a mother in the corner, but a deeper analysis would require a skillful, compassionate dissection. For months, only the superficial story remained. In the beginning, it became widely known that Chloe carried a diagnosis of bipolar disorder, and over time a crude portrait of her life and persona was painted. Soon the stigmatizations followed, in sweeping, abrupt, and insensitive characterizations of her supposedly compromised love for her daughter, her limited competence to provide ongoing care, and her absence from the bedside.

Chloe's daughter was hospitalized for nine months, and during one five-day period she was absent from the bedside. I heard the rumors flow down the hospital ward hallways.

"The mom is crazy."

"I bet she's lost her mind."

"She's never here anymore. Must have gone off her meds."

"How is she going to take care of this baby when she can't even take care of herself?"

As I was a human being with my own mental health story, it broke my heart to hear this whispered negativity. I wanted to know the proper truth of her story. Upon her return, I pulled out a chair and listened, sometimes for hours at a time, as we built a comfortable space that was safe enough for intimate disclosures.

The truth was that Chloe had a difficult life. She was abused at an early age, and struggled for several decades with post-traumatic stress related to her childhood experiences. She had been diagnosed with bipolar disorder only a few years earlier, and was working hard to navigate her mental health issues while tending to the myriad responsibilities of being a young single mother. The child's father had tragically died in an automobile accident while she was pregnant, only about six months before we first met. She didn't even have time to grieve before the next hit came: a fetal ultrasound and an uncertain future.

When she wasn't at the hospital, she was looking after her other child, working, or going to a multitude of appointments for her own health. She lived three hours away from the hospital, and finding transportation back and forth was difficult. Finances were tight, as she tried to save every last dime in preparation for her daughter coming home with complex medical needs. She wasn't crazy or off of her meds, and she wasn't being neglectfully absent from her daughter's life. She was a great mom, doing the best she could to manage difficult circumstances and take care of the ones she loved, which at times required taking care of herself.

Her daughter's surgery was important to reveal the true extent of her underlying disease, but dissecting Chloe's story proved to be a valuable moment of humanity, helping me understand her needs as well as those of her entire family. In order to preserve this humanity, I realized that it's necessary to start telling different stories. In my recovery, I learned to spend time listening with compassionate ears so that I can stand up to stigma when it confronts me head-on.

I meet patients' family members like Chloe every day, as well as colleagues who shudder when sharing their own mental health stories because of fear of the inevitable stigma. It is time that we start telling more accurate stories by listening closely for a more complete truth.

I learned to stop judging people by these superficial means and convenient characterizations. But I also learned that sometimes listening for this truth alone is not enough. Sometimes, standing up for another person is required.

Recently, when I heard a comment about a person being "nothing but a drug addict," I responded, "Awesome, me too."

What followed was a beautifully awkward thirty seconds of silence in which a new way of thinking was born, one to challenge the status quo of offhand comments.

I continued, "I wonder how they are doing in their recovery."

I was not being forceful or condescending, but rather trying to open their eyes to a world they may not have had any experience with. Inviting them into the dialogue and encouraging them to consider a fresh take on a tired old narrative worked. The same colleague came up to me a few days later and asked about my recovery, and then thanked me for sharing part of my story.

When a medical student presented a case during morning rounds, a cutting commentary of "Well, this patient is *really* schizophrenic" made its way into the summary of events.

After rounds, away from other people, I asked a follow-up question: "I was *really* depressed and suicidal once. How does that apply to the care we are giving this human being?" After a long silence came another moment in which eyes were opened.

Confronting stigmas with compassion, while taking the time to hear an individual's story, has allowed me to advocate for the truth of a narrative to find the light of day. In doing so, I can help to show Chloe's story through a different lens and promote a kinder, more accurate representation of her life.

I wasn't always that kind to myself. During my own struggles, and as a young child, I was the one being pushed down in the mud, not the helping hand pulling someone else back up. I didn't feel as though I was strong enough to get back up during those moments, nor did I feel worthy of doing so. I vowed that those events would never define my life, because my mental health story has made me stronger. And I promised myself I would not stand idly by when I see something like that happen to others.

Chapter Thirteen

The Vulnerability to Create Honest Conversations

On a Friday afternoon, my pager went off with a number I recognized from the pulmonary floor of the hospital. The caller, a bedside nurse, summoned me up to the pulmonary unit to have a chat with one of my patients.

She had been in the hospital for months when I stepped into her florally decorated room, which showed all the signs of her long stay—a teenager's hospital suite with computer screens, romance novels, an aromatherapy machine, and a makeup mirror on her bedside table. As I walked in, a Hallmark Channel holiday movie playing in the background provided a welcome ambience. I took a step closer to her bed, and she muted the Christmas bells with the TV remote. With a single finger, she waved me over to her bedside, and then motioned for me to sit down on the edge of the bed.

Her name was Lindsay, and she famously slept with a stuffed animal squirrel every night. She joked that the furry companion, which she named "Rocky," represented her tumultuous path. We sat briefly in silence as the hospital bed adjusted to absorb my weight, and she wiggled around to find a more comfortable position.

Then she said, "I saw something about you, and I wanted to talk to you about it."

"Okay, what's that?" I asked.

"I read online that you have a history of depression, and were suicidal once."

"Yes, that's true," I confirmed.

"That's pretty cool that you talk about it."

"Why do you say that?"

"Because I've felt that way too, but I never felt like I could talk to anyone."

"I didn't know that, Lindsay. Thank you for sharing."

"Well, I figured maybe you would understand."

She went on to say that she had struggled with depression for years, even before her long hospital stay, and in the past several months it had worsened. She added that she had thoughts of suicide, and had been cutting her legs for the past few months to "feel anything" amidst the growing pain in her life. She said she couldn't bring herself to tell anyone, not even her family. At first her head hung as she stared at the white linen sheets on her bed. For Lindsay, an inner shyness was forced to the surface by an underlying shame, so I listened patiently, without judgment, and let her express her truth.

As the conversation went on, her head lifted, and she even smiled in the realization that she wasn't alone in her feelings. She could talk about them with me and receive a compassionate understanding.

I thanked her for opening up, and we planned for a follow-up visit a few days later.

On my way out the door, she called me back to her bedside and leaned in to my ear.

She whispered, "Thank you."

For a brief moment, our vulnerabilities aligned in a deep connection of human understanding. Together, we created a space that could accommodate intimate details, because my own story gave her permission to speak openly about her truth.

However, for suffering individuals, honest conversations about mental health often stay closeted because of a lack of safe spaces in which to share.

I have now been on both sides of this issue—first, as an individual seeking treatment and navigating a broken system that discourages vulnerability and open communication; and second, as an agent seeking to bring forth cultural change that will carve out spaces for vulnerability and acceptance for colleagues, patients, families, and friends.

In my experience, the more vulnerability I show, the more opportunities I have to connect to other people. I learned the hard way that when I hide my true self from others, I spiral toward shame. Conversely, when I bury my shame, I begin to accept myself as a beautifully flawed human being, and my perspective on the world reflects that. A turn of the vulnerability dial has opened up connections to other people, while turning away pity, judgment, fear, and shame. Meanwhile, when I am able to create spaces for vulnerability, permission is granted to have open and honest conversations about mental health conditions on a larger scale. But I would never have learned these lessons without being humbled by this disease.

Yet culturally, the very idea of vulnerability is under attack. We are flooded on social media with images of perfect lives, where we rarely see anything other than highlight reels. More and more I feel we are boxing out authenticity—the unglamorous, the gritty, the setbacks, and the failures. We let fear of other people's opinions dictate our behaviors because of a culture that practices casual cruelty in argumentative, one-sided conversations. Putting our true selves out into the world now, in today's full-access society, allows the opinions of others to flood into our psyches. And these opinions rarely spark civil discourse. They merely embolden the expression of previously held beliefs, the casualty being the authenticity of the individual sharing a piece of his or her truth. In a shout-down society, with everyone on their own soapbox, it becomes easier to not say anything at all about the more difficult aspects of our lives. It takes true courage to speak authentic truth in modern society, because we constantly exist in a social-risk-reduction mind-set that is physically, emotionally, and spiritually exhausting.

With that idea in mind, I launched Malcolm Gladwell's podcast *Revisionist History* and listened to an episode titled "The Big Man Can't Shoot." In it, Gladwell recalled how, during the 1961–1962 NBA basketball season, Wilt Chamberlain averaged more than fifty points per game (50.4, to be precise). During that season, he completed his famous 100-point basketball game. In that game, Chamberlain shot thirty-two free throws, making twenty-eight of them, or 87.5 percent. In the prior year, he had been a 50.4 percent free-throw shooter, and during the season of his herculean 100-point game, Chamberlain raised his output to 61.3 percent.

The difference?

During that season, and during the 100-point game, Wilt shot his free throws underhand. This was a tactic made more mainstream by the Hall of Fame player Rick Barry in the 1960s and 1970s. Barry was a 90 percent career free-throw shooter, averaging 93.5 percent in his final year. This new tactic seemed to work for Wilt, as he was enjoying the greatest year of his career statistically. So, what happened next? Wilt returned to shooting the ball in the conventional overhand style, and his free-throw percentage dropped over the course of the next several years until it reached a career low of 38 percent in 1967–1968. Wilt had found a solution, improving upon one of the few weaknesses of his game, and the change in his approach was statistically rewarded—yet he simply stopped doing it. The theory here is that Wilt stopped shooting free throws underhand because it was not socially acceptable—it was a "granny shot," and he looked weak doing it. Simply put, Wilt abandoned something that worked for him out of a fear of breaking the cultural norms, a fear of being publicly vulnerable, and so he let other people's opinions dictate his behavior. It was a missed opportunity to embrace vulnerability, and in terms of statistical output, conforming to the norm hurt his career.

I have seen firsthand how the inability to be vulnerable comes at a great cost. Without the ability to open ourselves up, we lose the ability to take risks, forge new trails, fail, create, mature, and grow to understand true empathy with other people. How quickly we forget that some of the greatest advances in medicine originated either in repeated failures or by accident—warfarin, penicillin, the pacemaker, radiographs, Play-Doh, and the Slinky. (Okay, indulge me a bit on the last two; I work at a children's hospital, and both of those are an integral part of medicine.)

James Joyce once said, "Mistakes are the portals of discovery." Creative insight requires vulnerability, and that's the value you pursue as you risk making mistakes. These opportunities turned my life into a shotgun-riddled wall through which I now see a world opened up to future discoveries.

One of those mistakes turned into a grand lesson, as taught by a young couple fighting to save their son's life.

A few years ago, I was asked to attend a meeting in the hospital with the family of an infant with a complex medical diagnosis who was in a critical state. The meeting was supposed to take place a large conference room with a handful of medical professionals and the patient's parents. As the palliative care doctor, I was asked to tag along. Unfortunately, the meeting room was occupied and we had to find another location. When I showed up, there were ten people in a room about the size of a linen closet. The parents were sitting on a couch in the corner, three of the doctors were sitting in chairs, and the other seven were standing over the family in a circle. I barely made it inside the door. The family was literally backed into the corner farthest from the door, seemingly without any plausible route for escape. Breaking the bad news of the severity of the diagnosis came and went with a lot of medical jargon. The family sat there, did not ask any questions, and just like that, the meeting was over.

A few months later the dad called me into their son's hospital room to talk. He thanked me for my time, and expressed gratitude for our assistance over the last several months, but then asked if he could give some constructive feedback to the medical teams.

I said, "Absolutely, please do."

He said, "You know that meeting we had to talk about the diagnosis and what was going on with our baby?"

"Yes, I do remember," I replied.

"It was a really poor conversation. My wife and I both struggle with anxiety, and the team had us packed into a tiny room and seated in the corner. The situation was tense enough as it was, and with our heightened anxiety it felt out of control. We felt outnumbered, intimidated, and trapped. People were standing over us. It was hot. And there were people there we had not even met before. The tone and the terms made us feel as though we were being talked down to. I don't know how anyone could be expected to be open or vulnerable in a situation like that."

"You're right. We made a mistake. I'm truly sorry for that."

He was right; we had failed to create a space for an open, honest, and potentially vulnerable conversation. Without the proper environment, the rest is moot, and a conversation never happens; people just sit and lob words at each other.

My own experience in palliative care has given me a lot of insight into how to successfully communicate with others, and how to strategically construct environments and conversations. Having also lived through mental health recovery, I work to bring my experiences to bear in an effort to provide some framework for creating spaces that permit vulnerability and honest conversations regarding mental health conditions that affect our family, friends, colleagues, and patients.

In the field of palliative care, we often use the acronym "SPIKES" (Setting, Perception, Invitation, Knowledge, Explore Emotions, and Summary) in the context of sharing serious medical information with patients and their families, but it is really a template for having a successful conversation. Over time, I have applied this construct to the concept of holding spaces for individuals to speak about their own mental health conditions—patients, families, colleagues, and friends alike.

The "S" stands for Setting and is a reminder that the actual physical space is important to promote a safe arena for the expression of vulnerability. In the clinical setting, this means constructing a space that is not intimidating. The environment should include plenty of seats, a layout conducive to eye-level conversations, easy access to the door, ample room, and a limit on the number of individuals attending. Selecting the physical location is critically important as a first step to ensure a safe environment, yet inherent in the process is that attitude, tone, and language matter deeply too.

Not that long ago, I gave a talk about vulnerability in the workplace. I spoke of opening up an intimate environment for people to share their own truth about mental health conditions that have affected them personally or the people they love. A few days after the talk, a well-respected physician sent an email out to 100 people under his direction.

He wrote: "I just want to let everyone know I have a history of anxiety, I have been on medications successfully for many years, and I want to promote a culture where it is okay to seek help and treatment. You do not have to share personally; I just want you to know that my office is a safe space because I have been there too."

This email showed that vulnerability can be contagious and positive settings can be created. The trickle-down effect was that dozens of individuals reached out and sought treatment for their own mental health conditions. In the end, people felt empowered to share their stories, including some who have now taken a public stand. This approach is applicable not just in a medical context; it can happen in any workplace and in any setting.

Other positive environments can be created as well. Last year in our children's hospital, a team and I started a project called "Compassion Rounds," the purpose of which was to create safe spaces where all individuals working in the hospital could express feelings about the emotional difficulty of working in a place where children are sick and sometimes die. At every session, a panel of colleagues generously share their stories while hundreds of people sit in the audience in respectful silence. In every session, tears are shed, hugs are exchanged, and people learn more about the perspectives of people they pass in the halls every day. An environmental service worker spoke about the trauma of carrying a child down to the morgue for the first time, and a schoolteacher recalled reading a *Goosebumps* book at the bedside of a dying child. A surgeon talked about the grief he had felt after the unexpected death of a patient thirty years earlier. By sharing in these ways, we create settings, build community, forge connections, and open up pathways for human stories to find a safe and loving home.

The "P" is for Perception. In clinical palliative care, this simply means gaining an awareness of what the patient and/or family understands and what their perception is before beginning a dialogue. I start a meeting with a family by saying, "Tell me what the doctors have been telling you," or "Can you share with me what you know so far, in your own words?" The key is to not walk into these conversations with preconceived ideas—to shelve bias at the door—and to openly seek insight into another person's perception and perspective.

In recovery, I felt the effects of a lack of commitment to exploring this perception personally. I was willing to share my perspective openly, but the doors of empathic communication were sealed shut. When I met with a lawyer before appearing at the medical board to discuss my history of depression and alcoholism and to explain the depths of my underlying medical condition, the disconnection quickly became apparent.

I said, "I would love to share my—"

Abruptly, I was cut off. "I don't know how you don't think you'll be punished. You are an alcoholic doctor. We have to protect the safety of the patients."

I guess his mind was already made up.

So, I found a new lawyer.

With the new lawyer, I argued that the former lawyer's perception was flawed. I asked him, "What are the two most important things we can do to protect patient safety?"

"Not sure," he replied in a somewhat annoyed tone.

"Not working while sick, and washing your hands," I stated. "The problem with the first is that I am sitting in front of you defending my medical license because I openly admitted I was sick. At the same time, probably the most important thing a medical professional can do is wash their hands, but when someone fails to do so, they aren't brought in front of the medical board for punishment."

I took his simple nod as a small victory, and then went on.

"Protecting patient safety is critically important. But medical residents with untreated depression are six times more likely to make medication errors, so why don't we do anything and everything possible to get those doctors into mental health treatment? In truth, the oversight and litigation process for professionals with mental health conditions is not solely about the protection of patient safety at all, it is about maintaining the perception of it."

With his head down, he sighed. Then he slowly looked back up and said, "Looks like we have a lot of work to do."

The "I" is an Invitation statement. In palliative care, this means asking the patient and/or family for permission to have a sensitive conversation as a sign of respect and to give them control of the situation. I do not walk into a room and start saying, "So, your scans are back and the tumor has progressed." Sometimes, in the context of discussing mental health conditions in the workplace, this is exactly what it seems like. Conversations are often forced from places devoid of perspective, with an insensitivity to timing, a lack of proper context or setting, and without any input from the individual living with the condition.

I have been privileged to travel the country to speak and to meet countless individuals with their own mental health stories. When visiting one workplace, I found out that 46 percent of the employees had reported feeling distress in their jobs. I also learned that a member of the community had tragically died by suicide just a few months before my visit.

Out of good intentions, management's immediate reaction was to send out a survey to assess the risk factors associated with the ongoing levels of employee distress. In theory, this was an understandable attempt to get more information about the underlying causes of psychological distress in their workplace. But for the workers now grieving the loss of a colleague, the response to this approach was furious and swift.

From one individual I heard, "We just lost a friend and nobody is asking us how we are doing."

Another said, "Instead of being told to fill out a survey, why weren't we asked about what we need?"

The problem, as became abundantly clear, was that the survey was a strategic move executed in a bureaucratic mind-set that lacked any intent to invite the workers into a sensitive discussion. Many people felt it was poking the bear at the wrong time. No permission was asked; there was just an expectation to do more without any further explanation or discussion.

The "K" stands for Knowledge. In clinical terms, this means that having a difficult conversation requires that the medical professional be knowledgeable about the topic of discussion so that accurate and complete information can be shared during the encounter and then informed consent can be provided by the patient and/or family. The key is to avoid medical jargon and speak simply to the patient's level of understanding.

This also means that in framing conversations about mental health, leaders must educate themselves about the truth regarding mental health conditions. Rumors, falsehoods, fear, and rhetoric have run rampant for way too long. We need leaders who will educate themselves about the facts so that we can have productive conversations moving forward.

A few years ago, I attended a meeting in which policies regarding addiction in the medical workforce and the community at large were discussed. In one exchange, a local pharmacist made the statement, "Addicts are a substantial risk that must be mitigated in our hospital systems by a risk-management strategy." Ironically, many medical professionals are tragically undereducated about mental health and addiction conditions. We must stop the sweeping generalizations that lump individuals into stereotyped and stigmatized boxes, and move away from ignorant assumptions. Coming to the table with prejudices sets the conversation up for failure before it even begins. Leaders must acknowledge the presence of implicit biases and work to confront these biases head-on. The fact is that individuals with mental health and addiction histories work successfully every single day. The fact is that the number of people in the medical field who are working ill is shockingly large and growing at an alarming rate. The fact is that individuals working with untreated mental health conditions present a risk for work performance issues, yet avoid treatment for fear of stigmatization and punishment. The fact is that the culture we have created is a huge part of the problem.

The "E" is for Exploring Emotions. Clinically, this is about being present with your patients and walking with them during their journey without judgment or arrogant presumptions of knowing what it is like to experience what they are going through. It is simply about exploring another person's perspective and creating space for their emotional processing. In attempts to have successful conversations about mental health conditions, this is often where the ball is dropped.

When I told a coworker about my mental health recovery, his response was "I'm sorry. That sucks."

There were no questions, no explorations of how I really felt about the recovery process. The key is to never assume you know what someone else is going through, or what it means to them. When the colleague apologized to me, I thought, "Why is he sorry? This has been the greatest thing that ever happened to me."

When a young mother named Regina called me to the ICU bedside of her seven-year-old son, she asked if we could speak in another room, off the hospital floor. For several weeks our team had been caring for the boy while he remained critically ill from a progressive and resistant infection.

She said, "I was in recovery for six months, but I relapsed a few weeks ago from all the stress of what is going on."

I replied, "I appreciate you sharing with me; I feel honored. Do you mind telling me more?"

Regina said, "I just couldn't handle all of this. I didn't know what to do, so I fell back into old habits."

"I can't imagine what this has been like for you. How are you feeling?"

Then came a long silence. Her head fell into her hands, and she started to cry.

Without looking up, she said, "I just feel so alone."

She tapped her toes on the linoleum floor, in a moment of rising apprehension.

Then she lifted her head out of her hands and muttered, "Can you help me?"

"Of course. I'm here every step of the way," I told her.

Her head slowly raised from a downward gaze. I saw the expended tears in her eyes as she let out a sigh of relief.

"Thank you. You are the first person that genuinely asked me how I was doing."

The final "S" is for providing a Summary. In clinical medicine, this means taking a moment to ask the family to summarize a conversation to gain an appreciation of what they have understood from it. I ask families to use their own words and give a brief recap. The family might say, "We understand that our father is really sick right now, and the next days will be touch and go." Okay, the message was received. The second part is to articulate the next steps. In the patient scenario, I would listen to the summary and then say, "We'll meet again tomorrow to discuss it further," or "We'll perform some lab tests today and let you know the results." In the conversations about mental health in the workplace, this approach really revolves around transparency in the communication pathways between leadership and employees. There must be a clear, direct line of communication and feedback about institutional changes and about policies, programs, and initiatives that are in place to address the issues being discussed. Without an appropriate summary, the feedback loop is broken and the perception of any progress stagnates. The need for a good summary is critically important in larger workplace cultures that direct that timely feedback be provided to individuals in an appropriate forum. An appropriate summary can be simple: "I understand these are the major issues and barriers in our workplace, so we will form a task force and follow up in four weeks."

As someone who put this schematic into action, and was living an open and vulnerable truth about addiction and recovery, I was invited to have a seat at a larger policy table a few years ago. A task force was formed to pen an updated version of an addiction policy for an entire academic health system. Over the course of a year, dozens of meetings were held to rewrite the policy from scratch. The team was composed of lawyers, human resource officers, security personnel, hospital administrators, pharmacists, nurses, and physicians, and each of us was able to share our own experiences, our own biases, and our own feelings openly and honestly, in a safe space created for a productive conversation. We debated and disagreed, but respectfully afforded one another opportunities to share our personal perspectives. Two individuals with firsthand addiction experiences were not only invited to the table, but were given a voice and a direct say in the process. This was progress, and the final result was an astounding transformation of the health system's addiction policy—from one written only in a tone of bureaucratic, legal self-protection to one centering on human beings with treatable medical conditions. The opening line of the new policy was: "We recognize that individuals may be diagnosed with medical conditions, including mental health and addiction conditions, and our priority is to get these individuals treatment for these conditions." The policy goes on to extrapolate on the pathways of treatment in an empathetic tone that is intended to encourage individuals to seek out their own mode of treatment.

Getting a foot in the door to help change policy was a direct result of spending the previous few years of my life wearing a big, bold "A" on my chest with pride, not as a scarlet letter and not as an addict, alcoholic, or a person feeling ashamed. I wear the "A" as Adam, a human being with a story and a journey, and a man resolute and empowered by the struggles that define the lives of many of us. It was embracing vulnerability, opening an honest conversation, and then reframing the story in terms of strength and not weakness that made all the difference. I learned that vulnerability in an atmosphere of authenticity displays true strength.

Chapter Fourteen

Healing with the Art of Empathy

I aspired to work in medicine to help heal suffering. Then I became ill, and needed healing myself. In the depths of depression, I started to believe what I was once told by a professor at the beginning of medical school. He taught that maintaining a distance from the work was a tool for self-preservation, protecting a finite amount of career empathy that would constantly be depleted until there was nothing left to give. I was told that human connection drained the empathic well, and once it was dry, apathy, resentment, and brokenness followed. He and others taught a systematic form of coping with tragedy by desensitization. Every day, I see people who approach their life and work with a survivalist mind-set, wearing protective layers of emotional chain mail in an effort to deflect emotional arrows. And yet, day by day, I see those people tire under the weight of their ironclad shields.

I tried first to distance myself from the battlefield, then to desensitize myself with alcohol, and then to don heavy armor. Those strategies left me feeling empty, isolated, and without purpose. I couldn't run far enough away from the thoughts and feelings in my own mind, and being told to not feel them at all further invalidated me into the line of thinking that I was different from everyone else. Maybe I wasn't strong enough to be a doctor. Maybe I don't have what it takes. Maybe my personality conflicts with the steely, cold, detached demeanor required to be a successful medical practitioner.

In the depths of my soul, I always knew that teacher was wrong. I knew because I saw how loving my father was to his patients, such as when an eleven-year-old boy ran up to him at one of my first tee-ball practices. I saw my dad talk to that boy's parents then in a generous way that allowed him to be present for my practice, yet gracious to his profession. I overheard his kindness and patience on early Sunday morning phone calls, and I watched as he balanced those efforts throughout my childhood. In all the years I spent chasing esteemed mentors, famed institutions, and prestigious titles all across the country, I needed to travel on my own journey into darkness to see the light of healing flicker from a small town in southern Oklahoma and from the footsteps of my father.

Following in his example, I learned that empathy is not finite. I just had to connect it with a deeper meaning and purpose. In living through my experience, I now see in my own pain, suffering, and sadness resides a beauty, and an opportunity to help others. I learned that wounds become wisdom. And in the opportunity of my disease, this wisdom taught me that recovery, for all of us, is really about community, connection, and a greater sense of belonging.

In recovery, I switched careers to work in palliative care, a growing subspecialty in medicine with a focus on maintaining quality of life in the midst of life-threatening and/or life-limiting medical conditions. In this transition, I've been able to explore a more meaningful professional life, and I found an employer that values me for who I am. I joined an incredible team, surrounded myself with supportive people, set new boundaries, reset expectations, and together we continue to create safe spaces that allow for people to live their authentic truth. In these spaces, I see the power and privilege of working in medicine again, and the incredible opportunities to make an impact in other people's lives. In this environment, and with this new perspective, I learned to embrace the potential to care for other people in life and work, in order to live a much deeper and more fulfilling life.

I finally learned a way to extract the marrow of patient encounters while preserving the sanctity of my own sanity. In years of counseling and self-discovery, I learned how to balance empathy with the skills of a steady, trained hand, so that I could provide support to others in their struggles with a measured control. I could also bring that empathy with me in a way that allows me to live my own life and take care of my family.

For me, the greatest moments of reclaiming my humanity have come out of caring for individuals facing some of the most difficult times of their lives. This process has given me permission to explore the fragility of my own medical condition that was almost certainly life-limiting, as I discovered in the woods. I've lived through the fragility of life, stepping across lily pad islands of fractured pieces of my own mortality. My disease pressured me to confront the pointlessness of living another day. My professional duty affords me the opportunity to help other people answer their own questions about how to live each day well. As I do this work, often being invited into another person's story, a reciprocal healing takes place. I am blessed to be able to help other people navigate their own uncertain paths forward, and in doing so, I gain a profound gratitude for each day I am alive. When we are grounded in our mortality every day, it puts the rest of life into a greater perspective.

Allow me to share with you some of the stories of my patients and their families in order to show you how their narratives and experiences have gifted me with a greater sense of purpose in my own recovery process. These stories are not medical per se; they are tales of hope, loss, love, and kindness. They are human stories told within the context of medicine, but their significance extends into everyday life outside the hospital walls.

Let me tell you about a brave Maasai mother, about Louis, about Olivia, and about Nick. All are innately human stories that show the power of human connection. All have been critical points for me as I have traveled the path of my own recovery. I share them to inspire you to reach out to those you meet in your journey—to show up, be present, listen, and learn, no matter the expected outcome. In doing those things, I have learned that there is power in the journey, not just in what happens in the end. When we look at these kinds of experiences as daily steps in a journey, the power of empathy can mold any form of personal recovery into an exploration of deeper human connections.

Epiphany in Eldoret

I vividly remember a moment early in my recovery, while on a medical mission to western Kenya, when three colleagues and I walked up a hillside, out in the rural Maasai farmlands, a few hours from the city of Eldoret. It was monsoon season. The trek there required a seventy-minute hike due to rain-carved crevices on the sole access road. The mission was to deliver a mattress to a twelve-year-old boy with cerebral palsy who had spent most of his life sleeping on the dirt floor of his widowed mother's modest hut.

A beehive was nestled within an interior wall of their home, and I watched a mother walk out through a curtain of bees to greet us, a testament to her resilience. The boy lay on the floor due to his spastic immobility. I saw open sores on his back that must have been difficult to keep clean. Over the years his muscles had clearly wasted away, leaving a tensile battle of tendon versus bone. His skin was pulled tight like tissues of rubber bands, as the tension stretched him into unorthodox and uncomfortable positions. In what looked like a cruel discomfort, he smiled widely and his ears wiggled with his expanding grin. I saw how his short black hair was meticulously combed, and then turned around to see his mother sweeping the dirt floor with a homemade straw broom.

We had come to offer a small bit of assistance, the four of us hiking up the hillside while passing a mattress from one head to another and carrying handfuls of personal-care supplies.

Day in and day out, she carried her eighty-pound son on her back down the same roads. In the past, she had even carried him four hours each way on a fractured red clay road for a single trip to the medical clinic. Since the sudden passing of her husband, these trips had become increasingly difficult, as she had no one to help harvest their crops. Medicine was a distant luxury that her time and their mouths could barely afford.

We delivered the mattress, provided dressings, lotions, and ointments, and taught her techniques to stretch the boy's spastic limbs. They welcomed us into their home, and we shared an experience of true human connection in an atmosphere of overwhelming gratitude. I sat on the dirt floor, listening to our interpreter speak their Swahili dialect as the buzzing African bees hovered around our heads.

"Your gifts will be repaid in this life, or ever after," the mother said, placing her hands together in a prayerful steeple and gently nodding her head.

"Thank you for the blessing," our interpreter told her on our behalf.

"You are the blessings, my children. Travel well on your journey."

On the way back down the hill, I stopped. My colleagues were out of my sight. I took a deep breath, gazed over the canopy of brilliant, red-orange Nandi flame trees, and felt a great sense of inner peace. Ever since I had begun my career in medicine I had idolized the international aid work of Dr. Paul Farmer. I first read his story in Tracy Kidder's *Mountains Beyond Mountains*, and sadly felt I would never have the impact he had, as depicted in that book. Now at least I felt a little bit of resolve. By navigating a remote terrain, appreciating the beauty all along the way, to bring something meaningful to a person in need, I learned how to walk a mile in someone else's shoes, and it connected us all in a moment of profound joy.

Halfway down the hill, I looked down at the access road, and then glanced back over my shoulder at the young mother's hut. I saw every rock, every boulder, and every twist and turn in the path behind me. For a moment, instead of focusing on how much farther I still had to go to get to the car, I took stock of how far I had already come. I realized, step by step, that I was walking forward toward my own goals of personal recovery, and I had already overcome many obstacles along the way. Each rock, each boulder, and every twist and turn marked a milestone on my journey into a new life. I took a deep breath in, thankful I was exactly where I was supposed to be at exactly the right time. In the exhalation, I became overwhelmed by the incredible places my journey had taken me.

Louis's Goodbye

On a Friday evening in early April, one of my patients, Louis, came into the hospital. Louis was not just a patient; he was a mentor and an inspiration. On the same Friday evening, Louis was dying in his hospital bed from a rare, recurrent form of a cancerous lymphoma. Louis had a softly welcoming face, with ample cheeks and gentle green eyes. Under the shadow of his disease, the strength in his smile continuously shined, even while the tumors had spread and all therapies had failed to halt the progression of his cancer. In his final months, Louis enrolled in hospice treatment to maximize the quality to the remainder of his life. Louis truly lived during those months, traveling the country, speaking at churches, and inspiring other cancer patients with the occasional skydive out of an airplane. Then this beautiful twenty-three-year-old man came back to the hospital because he wanted to be with his friends at the end of his life—his friends being the nurses, doctors, therapists, and café staff he grew to love during two years of his on-and-off treatments.

I walked into his hospital room, sat down at his bedside, squeezed his hand one final time, and through trembling lips whispered, "I love you, brother."

His fingers squeezed mine in pulses that felt like Morse code for "I love you, too."

I looked up, a tear rolling down my left cheek, and his eyes confirmed that I had translated the code correctly.

Driving home, I reflected upon the fact that I had likely said my final goodbye to Louis. I was overcome by the sentiment that a young man had called me to his room to gift me with his presence during his final hours. How many people are blessed to be called to say goodbye? When moments are priceless and minutes are fading, to be invited into a sacred space. To deeply sense a person's light amid inaudible words, in the rhythm of unspoken air. I paused to inhale and to never let that moment go. There can be no assignment of value to that moment, nor can I ever adequately describe it with the written word. All I can tell you is that there is meaning and purpose within a genuine friendship, a love, a connection, and a bond that transcends the mortal gatekeeper's hand.

Today's customs and standards would say Louis's treatment was a failure—medicine failed him, and we failed him. But to simply label the end of Louis's life a failure diminishes his individual worth and discounts the greater meaning and purpose of his own journey, blinding us all to the impact that he had on other people's lives up to the very end. Is it heartbreaking that this beautiful, vibrant, articulate soul only lived to experience early adulthood? Absolutely. It is devastating and unfair beyond words. However, the quality of his life and the impact he had must not be undermined by quantitative measures, because as he told me himself, he did not want it that way.

Louis chose to focus on and measure the human impact, such as the impact the medical team had on him, and the gracious wisdom he imparted to us all during his remarkable life. He moved mountains of fear and anxiety for hundreds of other people through his outreach. He inspired thousands with online videos expressing hope and resiliency, and generously lived in his commitment to comfort others to his dying breath. His impact should be measured by his gift for helping children and young adults with cancer, teaching life lessons, and selflessly bestowing his enlightened perspective. He forever changed me, my colleagues, and other friends who walked the journey with him. The impact of such a life is world-changing.

In his final days, Louis told a young resident physician, "You have only one life," and then asked, "Now, how are you going to spend it?"

Instead of waiting for an answer, he then told the young doctor about a dream he had the night before of driving a white Mustang with black rims down the California coast—top down, sun on his face, wind in his hair. Louis didn't need an answer, I think he knew his lessons were complete.

Louis simply said, "I'm driving home."

Just a few nights before I wrote this page, and a few years after Louis passed away, the resident physician sent me a text message with a photo of a white Mustang with black rims, without any caption. I thought about the lessons that young man taught that young physician; how the doctor learned the meaning of living a life well.

I also thought of my own journey, and how Louis taught me to appreciate every day of my life as a gift. I simply smiled, then, imagining Louis cruising down the coast, free from tumors, IVs, and pain—driving home.

Showing Up and Paying Attention

A few years ago, I was consulted about a teenager with a complex history of a neuromuscular syndrome. The mother was nearing a crossroads where she would need to make difficult decisions about her child's medical care. A surgical intervention for her son's chronically dislocated hips was under consideration, among other possibilities. These were not necessarily life-or-death decisions, but they would certainly affect the child's life going forward, and she struggled to determine the right thing to do, as a lot of families do.

During that month, a medical student was rotating with our team. At this point, he had been with us for several weeks. I had been teaching him about exploring emotions, asking open-ended questions, and using empathic communication techniques. In our first meeting with the mother, we introduced ourselves as palliative care specialists and told her that we could assist her in weighing the potential risks and benefits of her impending decisions. We hoped we could help her solidify goals for her loved one's care. We noticed she was alone, and she told us that she did not have a lot of support.

The following day, we returned to continue the conversation and help her move forward in the decision-making process. But every time we broached the surgery option, it seemed like we hit a wall. We used exploratory questions such as, "Tell me more about what worries you."

She would say, "I just cannot see him on a breathing machine." (A ventilator would be required for surgery and post-op care.)

We kept hitting the same wall when asking follow-up questions, and would receive the same answer without further explanation. Insightfully, our student observed that the mother always wore the same large pendant necklace, emblazoned with a Christian emblem. When she spoke about not wanting to see her son on a ventilator, she held the necklace tightly in her hand over her heart.

The student asked, "I wonder if you could tell me about the meaning of your necklace."

The mother dropped her head and let out a deep sigh, and the tension fell out of her shoulders. She paused for a while, and we all sat in silence.

When she lifted her head, she spoke. "Three years ago, I was in a serious car accident with my brother and father in the car. My father died as a result of the accident. He spent the last three days of his life on a breathing machine in the hospital. And my brother was paralyzed. He spent seven months in the hospital because of his injuries. My mother and sister no longer speak to me—they blame me because I was driving, and I blame myself. That's why I'm alone. The last memory I have of my father is of him on that machine, so I just can't imagine seeing my son that way. This cross, my son, and my faith are all I have left."

She went on to share about her dark moments of depression, culminating in feelings of wanting to end her own life after the accident, in an all-consuming guilt. She said her son was the only reason she did not take her own life, and she couldn't imagine facing the demons she still carried if she ever lost him. Even just talking hypothetically about his death, she spiraled into moments where she felt like she was dying herself. And whenever someone wanted to talk about the surgery, she felt as though she was drowning in guilt for what had happened to her father and her brother.

Weeks of effort by other team members to obtain the mother's consent for surgery, and to explain the technical risks and benefits of the procedure, had not even scratched the surface of her burdens of fear, suffering, and anxiety. By being patient and observant, and by empathetically embracing the moment, the student and I were allowed to connect with her in a moment safe enough for her to reveal the true story behind her hesitation. It reminded me that we all guard our hearts, protecting intimacies of our past, and these secrets can weigh us down in isolation for the rest of our lives. I lived it myself in a different form, and hearing her story made that point of view seem perfectly understandable. I still don't pretend to know what her experience had been like, but I listened patiently so that I could try to imagine. I hope that in doing so I helped her realize she wasn't alone, as I realized I wasn't alone either in mine.

The Smallest Acts of Kindness

A few years ago, I opened up my work email at the end of a long work day. At the top of the queue was a name I recognized from my earliest days in medicine. With some apprehension, I opened the message to find a picture of a letter. Scribbled cursive on aged paper.

Her name was Olivia, and she was fifteen years old when we met. In her hospital bed, she sat in full knowledge of the gravity of the "C" word, but with teenage exuberance, she said that cancer should be scared of her.

Olivia had a quick wit, a sharp tongue, and no time for pretensions. She had short, curly brown hair, thinning from the rounds of chemotherapy, and a surgical scar running down the length of her left leg. Fresh into clinical medicine as a medical student working on the oncology floor, I drew the lucky straw to have Olivia as one of my first patients. After early-morning rounds, she quizzed me about the deeper meaning of *The Life of Pi*—a novel about a boy and a tiger stranded together in a lifeboat—with all its symbolism and allegory. We sat together as she ate pickles from a mason jar and the scent of vinegar wafted through the air.

"I didn't always like pickles, you know? Something about the chemotherapy and my taste buds. Suddenly, now I can't get enough," she said, taking another chomp.

With a wry smile, I weaved in some cursory medical questions about her nausea, vomiting, and comfort level during treatment. She tilted her head, placed her hands on her hips, and playfully said, "Just when I thought I could trust you! There you go, doctoring again."

She remained in the hospital for a few weeks of treatment, which was merely the beginning of the long journey ahead. As the days ticked by, we played cards, we talked about the transition to high school, and she shared some of her deepest worries and concerns about whether or not the chemotherapy would work. She trusted me, I admired her, and we built an indelible bond. On one of her final days in the hospital, I stopped by her room to say a friendly goodbye, but she was sound asleep. So, early in the morning, I left her a note on a scrap of paper in scribbled cursive, with a jar of pickles to hold it down.

"I hope you have a wonderful day. Enjoy the pickles. Maybe the tiger was really never in the boat, or maybe he was. Regardless, I know your boat is destined for safer shores."

Later that day, she was discharged from the hospital, I moved on to the next rotation, and we never saw each other again. Twelve years later, I scrolled through a pixelated email with a photographed letter and a brief note typed at the bottom of the screen.

I wanted to thank you for the kindness you showed me during
the toughest times of my life. My boat made it ashore. I still
have the letter, but I ate the pickles.

—Olivia

She didn't know it, but her kindness found me exactly when I needed it most. I've been privileged to share countless intimate moments with people during their struggles with illness. I understand what an incredible gift that is. Heartfelt rewards often flow from the mere fact of being present, and there is great power in those small acts of kindness we extend to each other every single day—moments often overlooked that actually change the world.

I barely even remembered writing that letter, and she kept it for twelve years.

It may have taken only five minutes of my day to pick up a jar of pickles and scribble a note, but to her it was poignant memento. The small gesture she returned over a decade later filled me with gratitude that I had made an impact on another person's life. In her act, she made me think about all of the small acts of kindness other people have extended to me, and how I need to spend more time telling those people about the positivity they brought me.

Her email changed the way I thought about medicine, and about the healing power of the smallest gestures of human kindness.

Nick's Gift of Love

In his short time on Earth, all Nick knew of life was cancer, having been initially diagnosed at the age of three. We met when he was fourteen. The latest iteration was a progressive sarcoma invading his spine, and he had come back to the hospital for another round of chemotherapy and radiation. Early in my career, only months into medical residency training, I was fairly sure I had an interest in oncology, but certain I had an interest in Nick. He was charming, charismatic, and kind, and he always cared more about other people than about himself. A young boy with an old soul, Nick spoke poetically in words of wisdom far beyond his years. For months, he cycled back through the hospital for treatments, but the cancer progressed. And yet his spirit remained. When his chemotherapy infusions were complete, I would visit him to pick up our friendship right where we left it off; I always tried to comfort him, yet he always seemed to comfort me.

In his final weeks, the tumor left him paralyzed from the waist down and confined to a bed. I vividly remember writing the orders for his pain medication drips and thinking the Drug Enforcement Administration could arrest me on the spot for prescribing such huge doses of Dilaudid. The DEA did not come, though, and the meds helped. He still endured pain, but he continued to comfort all those around him anyway. His mother was a nurse at the hospital, part of the lifeline helicopter crew, and toward the end of his journey she and her husband made the decision to take him home so he could spend the precious little time he had left with his family.

A week later, I received a phone call. On the line was the receptionist in the oncology clinic. "Nick is here. He did not want to talk to anyone else. He came to see you."

I paused for a moment, and said I would be right down. I grabbed a notepad and an envelope from the call room table, and I sat, took a breath, and wrote a note, crying as I signed it.

The contents are for him and his family, but the essence is that I told him how much I loved him, how proud I was of him, and how much he had changed my life. I folded up the note, fumbled it into the envelope, and headed down the stairs. As I came around the corner, his mother and father were standing there, and they began to cry. His mother said, "He told us this morning he still had one last thing he had to do." They opened the curtain to usher me into his room, and then closed it behind us. While it was clear that Nick was physically dying, his spirit was still savoring every moment. We sat, shared, laughed, and cried. I told him how the lessons he taught me had made me a better man and a better doctor, and in that moment, in his pain, he thanked me. I hugged him and slipped him the note, and after an hour we said goodbye. I remember feeling inadequate for having learned some of the greatest lessons of my life from him. It was like I had taken away more than I was able to give.

The next day, a Saturday, Nick passed away. His mother called me to say that she was reading the note I had written for him when he passed. "I told you, he had one last thing he needed to do—he needed you to know how much he cared about you." I still feel inadequate in telling his story, and unworthy of the gifts he gave me—yet that was Nick, selfless to the very end. His actions serve as a shining example of caring for others with every single breath and enjoying the gift of every moment. When we in medicine lift the veil of pretense, drop the walls of separation, and shed the white coats, people like Nick teach us all that we can heal each other. He cared about me, I cared about him, and that matters deeply. Nick taught me that love is the greatest reward for a job well done in caring about another person's pain and suffering. I didn't earn it; he gave it to me. But he taught me how to show up to receive it.

With Patience, the Real Story Will Emerge

I will share one last story about empathy in palliative care, an experience that illuminates the trust required to be invited into personal places. I had the honor of working with a family of a critically ill child, a family that had been in the hospital for several months as they watched their infant son get sicker and sicker from a rare genetic condition. It became clear to the medical team that this child would not survive his stay. There were no treatments or cure options, only the choice to prolong his life by artificial means.

For weeks, the medical team worked with the family, comforting them in their processing of an evolving tragedy. I met the family weeks into their journey and started to build a relationship with them. I started simply by getting to know them and their support structure, and scratched the surface of the story of their lives. Over time our rapport grew stronger, but then I sensed them backing away. In the stages of grief, they had cycled through denial and anger and were stuck in bargaining for more time with their loved one. Sometimes, a "clinical visit" consisted of simply bringing them a soda or dropping off a note to say I was thinking about them—not forcing the issue, but respecting them and their space while continuing to let them know I cared.

A few days later, the father called me up to the room, where I was invited into their private space. His soft-spoken wife sat in a bedside chair while he somberly paced from corner to corner. I offered a casual introductory sentiment, and he turned away, put his head in his hands, and cried. I reached over, put my hand on his shoulder, and acknowledged his emotions while I explored the meaning behind the tears.

"I can see that you're going through a hard time. Do you mind sharing what happened?"

A few moments passed, and then he turned to me and said, "I just can't go through this again."

I sensed a seismic shift happening, yet as I stood there, I did not know direction it was taking.

Softly, I asked, "Could you tell me more about that?"

The father explained that several years earlier, in a previous marriage, he lost a child.

"We had to make the decision to take her off life support," he said with a deep exhale. He was holding back the urge to weep. "I just can't go through that again."

All this time, in the months of discussions I had with these parents, it had never been revealed that this heartbroken man was struggling with the lingering effects of bereavement and post-traumatic stress disorder (PTSD) from the death of another child who was hospitalized. It was only then, after many weeks, many acts of kindness, and hours and hours of trust building to create a supportive space, that he was ready to disclose his story.

Of course his unfathomable loss had directly impacted the way he viewed the world, the decisions he would make, and his own behavior, forever. Acknowledging this prior tragedy, and then taking time to process the newly triggered emotions, was necessary before he could move forward in dealing with the events unfolding before his eyes. At the same time, the mother was suffering from the thought of losing her firstborn child, while also not knowing how to help her husband through the difficulties he was expressing.

This family's story was deeper than any preconceived notion could have captured, and it was not until that story was cautiously delivered and empathetically heard that they were able to move forward. I witnessed their heartache, and while I couldn't change it, I was present in a sincere way, and stepping into that process with them brought us close together in a connection of the truest form.

I learned the deeper meaning of standing with a family during difficult times when I was a patient myself. Those months taught me a new way to practice medicine. Instead of hiding my truth, I decided to use it to help guide others, because the art of empathy is in embracing our humanity, not hiding behind it. Empathy resides in walking a long, fractured clay road in another person's shoes, and in the wisdom gifted by a young man at the end of his life. It is about showing up, being patient, and partaking in small acts of kindness. The true art of empathy is to let yourself feel, and be moved by the compassionate love required to care for another human being.

In embracing the art of empathy, medicine has an extraordinary opportunity to heal. Because when it is all said and done, medicine heals when one person dedicates their time to earnestly listen to another person's story.

I sincerely thank you for taking the time to listen to my story. I hope you will find a place of safety to tell yours as well. I hope we can all feel empowered to stand up for other people who feel bullied or judged due to the struggles in their lives.

For me, I know my children are watching, without any preconceptions, labels, prejudices, or discriminatory notions. In their simple view of the world, there is joy in being able to connect to other people. When they get home from school, they just want a listening ear and a safe place to tell their story.

I hope to keep it that way.

Acknowledgments

My life, my career, and this book wouldn't be possible without my wife, Lauren, and her unwavering love and support through some the most difficult trials life can offer. To my parents, Mark and Marigay, who sacrificed so much to support their son. My sister, Amanda, who loves unconditionally with an open mind and loving heart. For our children, Grayson and Zoe, for giving me a reason every single day to be a better man and father. To all of my extended family for their kind words of continuous encouragement. To my closest friends, Graham, Justin, and Chuck, who stuck by me without judgment and always offered up a listening ear. To Jessica, Kristin, and Ray: your friendship, love, and support through the darkest times will never be forgotten. To Shannon and Kristin for being the first people to read this book, and giving me the encouragement to see it all the way through. To my palliative care work family: Amy, Caitlin, Amy, Karen, Kari, Becca, Kelli, Shannon, and Mona—you gift me a safe space to be my authentic self every day and I am grateful. To my bosses, Dr. Elaine Cox, Dr. Marie Cole, Dr. Jerry Rushton, Dr. Paul Haut, Dr. Lyle Fettig, Dr. Greg Gramelspacher, Dr. Wade Clapp, Dr. Greg Sachs, and Jim Luce—thank you for opening up your minds and hearts to support a young professional looking for a career home. And to my agent, Linda Konner, for taking a chance on an unknown author and helping me find a platform to tell my story.

To all my counselors and the recovery community who continue to help me stay sober one day at a time.

To Luke, Nick, Zoe, and all of my patients and their families for graciously allowing me to take care of them during some of the most difficult times of their lives.

For support of my lectures and this book I also would like to sincerely thank the following: Dr. Jamilah Hackworth, Dr. Derek Wheeler, Dr. William Considine, Dr. Michelle Howenstine, Dr. Sarah Friebert, Laura Pickard, Akron Children's Hospital, Cincinnati Children's Hospital, Community Health Network, Indiana University Health Physicians, Indiana University School of Medicine Graduate Medical Education, Choctaw Medical Center, Saint Louis University, and Butler University.

Finally, to my community at Riley Hospital for Children. This book wouldn't have been possible without all of you giving me the courage to be myself. Thank you to the greatest children's hospital in the world and a place that always makes me feel like I'm home.

Notes

1. Center for Disease Control (CDC). "Suicide Rising Across the US" www.cdc.gov/vitalsigns/suicide/infographic.html, accessed June 7th, 2018.

2. "QuickStats: Suicide Rates for Teens Aged 15–19 Years, by Sex - United States, 1975–2015." *MMWR Morb Mortal Wkly Rep* 66 (2017): 816 https://doi.org/10.15585/mmwr.mm6630a6.

3. VA Benefits & Health Care Utilization Pocket Card, Updated 5/13/16; Produced by the National Center for Veterans Analysis and Statistics www.mentalhealth.va.gov/docs/2016suicidedatareport.pdf

4. American Foundation for Suicide Prevention. *Facts about physician depression and suicide.* http://www.afsp.org/preventing-suicide/our-education-and-prevention-programs/programs-for-professionals/physician-and-medical-student-depression-and-suicide/facts-about-physician-depression-and-suicide.

5. Shanafelt, Tait D. "Changes in Burnout and Satisfaction With Work-Life Balance in Physicians and the General US Working Population Between 2011 and 2014." *Mayo Clinic Proceedings* 90, no. 2 (n.d.): 1600–1613.

6. Gold, Katherine J. "I Would Never Want to Have a Mental Health Diagnosis on My Record: A Survey of Female Physicians on Mental Health Diagnosis, Treatment and Reporting." *General Hospital Psychiatry*, September 2016. https://doi.org/10.1016/j.genhosppsych.2016.09.004.

7. National Institute of Mental Health (NIH). Mental Illness. 2017 National Survey on Drug Use and Health. https://www.nimh.nih.gov/health/statistics/mental-illness.shtml

8. World Health Organization. Health Topics: 2019 Depression Statistics http://www.searo.who.int/india/topics/depression/about_depression/en/

9. Mata, D. "Prevalence of Depression and Depressive Symptoms Among Resident Physicians: A Systematic Review and Meta-Analysis." *JAMA*, 2015. https://doi.org/10.1001/jama.2015.15845.2383-2373:(22)314,2015.

10. Rotenstein, LS, MA Ramos, and M Torre. "Prevalence of Depression, Depressive Symptoms, and Suicidal Ideation Among Medical Students: A Systematic Review and Meta-Analysis." *JAMA* 316, no. 21 (2016): 2214–36. https://doi.org/10.1001/jama.2016.17324.

11. Cohen, Deborah. "Medical students with mental health problems do not feel adequately supported: Survey provides a snapshot of mental health problems among medical students in the UK." ScienceDaily. ScienceDaily, BMJ. 1 September 2015. www.sciencedaily.com/releases/2015/09/150901204813.htm.

12. Sen, S, HR Kranzler, and JH Krystal. "A Prospective Cohort Study Investigating Factors Associated with Depression during Medical Internship." *Arch Gen Psychiatry* 67, no. 6 (2010): 557–565.

13. "More than 80% of Medical Students with Mental Health Issues Feel under-Supported." *Student BMJ Survey, Student BMJ*, September 2015, 34–36.

14. Starr, Kristopher T. "The Sneaky Prevalence of Substance Abuse in Nursing." *Nursing* 45, no. 3 (March 2015): 16–17. https://doi.org/10.1097/01.NURSE.0000460727.34118.6a.

15. Monroe, TB, H Kenaga, MS Dietrich, MA Carter, and RL Cowan. "The Prevalence of Employed Nurses Identified or Enrolled in Substance Use Monitoring Programs." *Nurs Res* 62, no. 1 (2013): 10–15.

16. National Alliance of Mental Health. National Mental Health Facts in America https://www.nami.org/NAMI/media/NAMI-Media/Infographics/GeneralMHFacts.pdf

17. Berge, Keith. "Chemical Dependency and the Physician." *Mayo Clinic Proceedings* 84, no. 7 (2009): 625–631. https://doi.org/10.1016/S0025-6196(11)60751-9.

18. Skutar, C. "Physicians Recovery Network Targets Attitudes about Impairment." *Mich Med* 89, no. 12 (1990): 30–32.

19. Kliner, DJ, J Spicer, and P Barnett. "Treatment Outcome of Alcoholic Physicians." *J Stud Alcohol* 41, no. 11 (1980): 1217–1220.

20. Gallegos, KV, and M Norton. "Characterization of Georgia's Impaired Physicians Program Treatment Population: Data and Statistics." *J Med Assoc GA* 73, no. 11 (1984): 755–58.

21. Brooks, E, M H Gendel, D C Gundersen, S R Early, R Schirrmacher, A Lembitz, and J H Shore. "Physician Health Programmes and Malpractice Claims: Reducing Risk through Monitoring." *Occupational Medicine* 63, no. 4 (June 2013): 274–80. https://doi.org/10.1093/occmed/kqt036.

22. Dijamco, Cheri. "Staying Sane: Addressing the Growing Concern of Mental Health in Medical Students." American Medical Student Association. 2015. https://www.amsa.org/2015/09/08/staying-sane-addressing-the-growing-concern-of-mental-health-in-medical-students/

23. World Health Organization. "Investing in mental health." Mental Health Update Statements. Accessed June 29, 2012. https://www.who.int/

24. Himmelstein, David U, Robert M Lawless, Deborah Thorne, Pamela Foohey, and Steffie Woolhandler. "Medical Bankruptcy: Still Common Despite the Affordable Care Act." *American Journal of Public Health* 109 (2018): 431–33. https://doi.org/10.2105/AJPH.2018.304901.

25. Hughes, P H, N Brandenburg, and D C Baldwin Jr. "Prevalence of Substance Use among US Physicians." *JAMA* 267, no. 17 (1992): 2333–23339. [published correction appears in *JAMA* 268, no. 18 (1992): 2518]

26. McLellan, A T, G S Skipper, M Campbell, and R L DuPont. "Five Year Outcomes in a Cohort Study of Physicians Treated for Substance Use Disorders in the United States." *BMJ* 337 (2008): a2038.